THE
CARBOHYDRATE
APPROPRIATE
DIET

ALSO BY CLIFF HARVEY

Time Rich Practice
Time Rich Cash Optional
99 Things You Need to Know to Lose Fat!
Choosing You!

CO-AUTHOR

Low Carb in Practice
(Simon Thornley, Peter Bowden and Cliff Harvey)

THE CARBOHYDRATE APPROPRIATE DIET

GO BEYOND LOW-CARB DIETS TO LOSE WEIGHT FAST AND IMPROVE ENERGY AND PERFORMANCE, WITHOUT COUNTING CALORIES

CLIFF HARVEY

KATOA HEALTH PUBLISHING | AUCKLAND, NEW ZEALAND

Published by Katoa Health Publishing (CC Publishing), a division of CC
Industries Ltd.
7 Ascension Place, Rosedale, Auckland 0632, NZ
Visit our website at www.KatoaHealth.com

ISBN 978-0-9941313-2-4
First Edition

Dedicated to the pioneers in the field of lower-carbohydrate nutrition—Drs Atkins, Volek, Phinney and Di Pasquale, and the renegades Dan Duchaine and Lyle McDonald. You were the voices that set me on this path all those years ago.

And to David 'Devo' Walden.
You pushed me to be a better version of myself mate, and you encouraged me to keep on pushing.
Hooley Dooley! Hold the phone!
It was, and remains one hell of a ride.
Miss you every day Padrino.

CONTENTS

TABLES & FIGURES

FOREWORD BY PROFESSOR GRANT SCHOFIELD

I'd spent the better part of a decade wondering what Cliff was on about. I was preaching conventional wisdom around nutrition and lifestyle.
Cliff was talking about eating more fat and less carbs.
For goodness sake, this was exactly the opposite of what we were doing…

There is an old story about a young man recounting (now that he is 21 years old) how he is surprised just how much more sensible his father has become over the past five years. He says "five years ago he was making no sense at all, but he's really grown up and learned lots".

Of course, it's easy for all of us, especially if you are a parent yourself, to see that it is the boy who has 'grown sensible' and finally has the maturity to understand the wisdom of his father…

The same story is one I can tell you about Cliff Harvey. I'd spent the better part of a decade wondering what Cliff was on about. I was preaching conventional wisdom around nutrition and lifestyle. Cliff was talking about eating more fat and less carbs. For goodness sake, this was exactly the opposite of what we were doing. Frankly, we thought Cliff was a bit nutty. As Cliff puts it he has been "out in the wilderness for so long", and that's true literally and figuratively.

I've been surprised how far Cliff has come in the last few years. Actually, on closer inspection, he's pretty much saying the same sensible, scientific stuff. It's me and my team that have grown up in the last few years. So it's with great pleasure that I have been able to get involved in working with Cliff as part of our team at the Human Potential Centre. We've learnt so much from him and will continue to for some time. The irony now, of course, is that Cliff is studying for a research degree in nutrition under my supervision (he aims to eventually complete his Ph.D.). Hopefully, I will know a bit more about the research process and can provide some guidance there!

It's also a pleasure to write the foreword in a book where personalized nutrition around carbohydrate restriction is the key concept and element. I love the idea of carb-appropriate nutrition. It's time to move beyond a "one size fits all" diet plan. Cliff shows us that we can (and should) adjust our carbohydrate intake depending on our biology and goals. He does this is in the context of eating whole, real food and backs everything with fully referenced scientific evidence.

Carb-appropriate nutrition is a diet book. It guides you on how to decide for yourself what and how you should eat. But importantly it doesn't stop there, he covers the other essential strands of living well – sleeping, mindfulness and exercise. Amongst all of this are some great practical tips for coping with "nutritionally challenging times and situations", like when you come home from work stressed, or when you feel like something sweet near bedtime. I personally got a lot from reading this book and hope you do too.

Grant Schofield Ph.D.

March 2016.

INTRODUCTION

A RETURN TO REAL FOOD

Why did it become so controversial to recommend whole and unprocessed, real food?

I've often wondered when it became so controversial to promote diets based on real food? And why is it seen as an extreme measure to use nutrition strategies that are appropriate to our collective evolution as a species, that are part of our collective heritage, and that are also culturally appropriate?

Thankfully what was once fringe is (re-) entering the mainstream, and lower-carbohydrate nutrition is now finally recognised for its considerable clinical value. But this isn't a book about low-carb nutrition, it's a book about how to find *your* unique template for nutrition based on nearly two decades of clinical application and research.

I coined the term 'Carb-Appropriate™' nutrition many years ago. This term, and the concept of nutrition it describes goes beyond low-carbohydrate nutrition for-all and delves into what is appropriate for the individual. There is, after all, a large range of carbohydrate tolerance amongst individuals. Many of us benefit from much lower carbohydrate intakes than those prescribed in the medical and dietetic mainstream, but there are also people who thrive at the higher levels of carbohydrate intake (Google 'Banana Girl' for an example!)

The Carb-Appropriate method allows clinicians, athletes, coaches and the public to understand better what their unique carbohydrate (and fat and protein) requirements are for their desired goals.

The foundation of Carb-Appropriate is a return to real-food nutrition. Most of us know intuitively that whole, unprocessed, unrefined foods help us to feel, look and perform at our best. Research is beginning to prove the ease with which people can improve their health and performance by eating a diet that based on a compendium of natural, whole and unprocessed foods—without the need to fastidiously count calories and macronutrients. This strategy is in stark contrast to the 'starvation and deprivation' mind-set of the typical calorie-restricted diet, and the treadmill obsessed 'burn it off' exercise strategies that have become the norm in best-practice guidelines.

We need a return to real food, primal movement, play, challenge, and relaxation and mindfulness. I hope this book will provide some of the tools you can use to improve your health and performance.

ACKNOWLEDGEMENTS

To all my friends and family, spread around the world and too numerous to mention, you know who you are. I love you all.

I t was becoming increasingly frustrating to be 'out in the wilderness' for so long, and thus, it has been an enormous boost to have been joined on this real-food, lower-carb journey by my colleagues at AUT University. Thanks to Professor Grant Schofield, Eric Helms, Dr Mikki Williden, Dr Caryn Zinn, Joe McQuillan, Dee Holdsworth-Perks, and Dr Nigel Harris and Dr Simon Thornley for your continued support and friendship. Thanks especially to Eric, Caryn, Grant, Sol Orwell, Dr John Berardi and Philip Dowling for reading the drafts, giving feedback, and challenging me to make the changes necessary to make this a better book and me a better author and researcher.

Colin, Duncan, Jason and Amber you have been there on this nutrition and science ride since the very beginning. Ian Brooks—thanks for getting me started on this whole writing lark (six books later!)

Without the help and support of my team at the Holistic Performance Institute; Emily, Kerry, Kate, Maria,

Sridhar, Carolyn, Kirsten, Laura, and all of our amazing members and colleagues none of this would be possible.

Pete Rive deserves special mention for always being able to read my mind to create amazing book covers and images. I'm blessed to have an artist of his stature on-call!

My friend and solicitor Simon Cogan, thanks for having my back homie.

Everyone at NuZest especially Trevor and Monique Bolland, Jonny and Aimee Edwards, Michael Lavender, Geoff, Claire and the Ashenden clan, and the NuZest NZ team.

Charlene, Dad, Kent, Bella, the Waldens and my extended family, who are always there to support and guide me.

Thank you.

I love you all.

CHAPTER 1

INAPPROPRIATE BEGINNINGS

Bro science & getting kicked out of nutrition class

My journey in nutrition began somewhat inauspiciously. I found myself on a hot, stuffy summer's afternoon sitting in the Dean's office of the college I was attending.

"Your conduct in class is disruptive. You've done enough to pass the course, and so your attendance is no longer necessary..."

I was getting kicked out of nutrition class!

With these fateful words my good friend Andrew and I were saved from the boredom (punctuated by frustration) that was our nutrition lectures. I know what you're thinking...I must have been a bad student, recklessly disrupting the learning of others in the class, but in truth, I was simply asking inconvenient questions. You see what we were being taught all those years ago just didn't make any sense! On the one hand, we were taught fairly self-evident truths of the anatomy and physiology of the human body and on the other nutrition concepts that stood in stark contrast to those roles.

In college, we learn the roles of the macronutrients (carbohydrate, protein and fat) that make up the diet. We learn that the amino acids that make up the protein we eat are the 'building blocks' of the body, and thus, protein provides for the structure of cellular components, cells, tissue, organs and the systems that these make up in the body. These amino acids also provide the building blocks for neurotransmitters (chemical messengers) such as epinephrine, norepinephrine, melatonin, serotonin and dopamine.

We learn that fat also provides building material for various cell components (including much of the brain and the phospholipid membrane around cells) and the various steroid hormones (e.g. testosterone, oestrogen, progesterone, cortisol, DHEA, androstenedione, and others). Fat, of course, is also a primary fuel and provides most of our energy at rest and lower levels of exercise activity.

And so we can simplify the roles of the macronutrients as:

1. Protein = STRUCTURE
2. Fat = STRUCTURE & FUEL

But what is the role of the third macronutrient, carbohydrate?

The major role for almost all carbohydrate in the body is fuel, and while it also has some very important (for example signalling) roles in conjunction with protein as 'glycoproteins', it is almost exclusively an energy providing macronutrient. And so to add to our simplified definitions above we can add:

3. Carbs = FUEL

Imagine my surprise that having learnt these concepts we were subsequently instructed in nutrition class that a *minimum* of 65% of people's calories should come from carbohydrate, irrespective of condition or state of activity. To me, this didn't stack up.

I peppered the lecturers with questions such as *"But what if someone is really sedentary, surely they don't need that much FUEL?"… and "How can someone wanting to retain muscle while dieting consume the optimal amount of protein (as indicated in the literature) if they have to eat 65% carbohydrate?"*

As you can probably guess it was these types of questions that led to the visit to the Dean's office and subsequent banishment from nutrition class.

I have to admit I wasn't overly worried by my exile as it provided the freedom to a) do more surfing and b) to delve more and more deeply into lower-carb strategies for nutrition. It was frustrating though to not have any intelligent answers or even meaningful discussion around the questions I was posing.

My continued exploration of low-carb around this time was (I am confessing my sins here) via bodybuilding magazines like M*uscle Media 2000*, *Ironman* and *Testosterone* that we might now call 'bro-science'. I'd now look back on those as less than stellar scientific references, but they had an excellent line-up of contributors who were scientist-cum-practitioners. Many of these contributors went on to become renowned in the fields of protein metabolism, low-carb nutrition and supplementation. One name that stood out (probably because he was most definitely NOT a researcher or practitioner) was Dan Duchaine, author of *Underground Body Opus.* While not being a researcher Dan was, in my opinion, one of the foremost minds in the emerging low-carb field. In those early days of my practice, use and prescription of lower-carb diets, his book *Body Opus* was a veritable bible.

On reflection, I have to thank my early lecturers for their curmudgeonly attitudes and our Dean for allowing us that extra (self-directed) study time! If not for that I'm sure I wouldn't have blazed off in a different direction into unknown territory, *lower-carb territory*. More importantly, I wouldn't have had the blessing of helping many thousands of people to live healthier, happier lives, with improved performances through a shift to a more pragmatic style of nutrition than that offered by the dogma of *thou shalt eat high carb*.

CHAPTER 2

WHERE DID WE GO WRONG?

Low-fat guidelines, sky-rocketing obesity
& diabetes

To anyone with eyes to see it is apparent that our current ways of eating are not serving us.

We have rapidly increasing rates of diabetes, a growing obesity problem and a worrying trend towards the pre-diabetic states that we categorise under the heading 'metabolic disorders'. We are also now beginning to understand better the role that poor metabolic health plays in the causation and progression of other non-communicable diseases such as cancer, heart disease and neurological disorders (which together are the leading causes of mortality and morbidity in the developed world).

For a long time now I have campaigned for a real-food based approach to nutrition, and one that includes low- and lower-carbohydrate nutritional strategies for the many people that would benefit from their use. I have been joined in this endeavour over the last few years by several prominent academics, researchers and clinicians who, as the weight of scientific evidence has mounted, have begun to believe that our current dietary guidelines for health are outdated and need drastic revision.

RAMPANT OBESITY, DIABETES AND METABOLIC DISORDER

The obesity rate in the United States in 2010 was 35.5% among adult men and 35.8% of adult women.[1] In my home country of New Zealand, perceived to be a bastion of 'clean green' living and physical activity, the current rates of combined obesity and overweight stand at around 65% of the population[2]…That's right, in the land of the All-Blacks nearly 2/3 of people are now either overweight or obese.

In 2011, there were 366 million people worldwide with diabetes, and this is expected to rise to 552 million by 2030.[3] The trend towards obesity and diabetes is being mimicked by nearly every country in the world, and these figures are steadily rising in spite of public health initiatives to improve diet and increase activity.

It has been estimated (based on the cost to life-expectancy of obesity related disorders[4]) that life-expectancy may level-off or drop for the first time in developed nations over the first half of the 21st century.[5] This will serve to reduce the positive effects of population life-expectancy from reduced rates of smoking[6] and will for the first time begin to undo the large increases in lifespan that have been achieved through the advent and development of improved surgeries, pharmaceuticals and reduced mortality due to vaccine-preventable deaths. We could be the very first generation to live a shorter lifespan than our parents in spite of all the amazing medical advances and greater awareness of health that we now have—and we are undoing all that good work through poor diet and lifestyle choices.

If these estimates are indeed correct, we have to ask ourselves *"Are the current guidelines for nutrition, simply not being followed? Or are they fundamentally flawed?"*

ARE OUR DIETARY GUIDELINES FOR HEALTH PARTIALLY TO BLAME?

One of the myths that public health departments sell us is that the dietary guidelines are sound and that if people only followed them, we would see reductions in obesity and diabetes (and the other disorders in which metabolic dysfunction plays a role). But when I speak to other practitioners the overwhelming feeling is that people are trying to follow the guidelines and are succeeding in following them (at least partially or wholly) and in spite of their best efforts are still becoming increasingly overweight, fatigued and sick. In my time in clinical practice, I have not seen people wantonly ignoring this health advice. On the contrary, I see people trying to eat 'low-fat' and 'low-sodium', 'low-calorie' foods and trying diet-after-diet to stay in shape! More often than not they are confused and frustrated because in spite of their efforts they are not able to get the results they desire. According to the Centres for Disease Control 'National Health and Nutrition Examination Survey' (NHANES)[7] average calorie (energy) intake per day has risen in spite of the recommendation to reduce fat to reduce calories (a flawed rationale that we will examine in greater depth later). (Figure 1.)

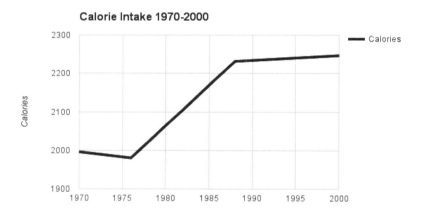

Figure 1. Total Energy Intake. Adapted from NHANES data.
http://www.cdc.gov/mmwr/preview/mmwrhtml/mm5304a3.htm#fig1

Data from NHANES indicates that the recommendation to reduce fat intake and prioritise carbohydrate *IS being followed* as seen in Figure 2. Intake of fat has fallen, as has that of the unfairly demonised saturated fats, while carbohydrate intake has risen. Overall calories have increased, and fat-gain and metabolic disorder have also concurrently increased.

[16]

So we are following the guidelines to eat less fat to help us eat less total calories (less fuel), and yet that has seen us eating a greater total of calories. Therefore, it's not surprising that there has been a fairly drastic increase in rates of diabetes and obesity across all age groups.

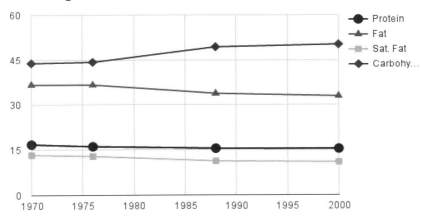

Figure 2. Protein, Fat, Saturated Fat and Carbohydrate Intake as a % of Calories. Adapted from NHANES data.
http://www.cdc.gov/mmwr/preview/mmwrhtml/mm5304a3.htm#fig1

As my students know well, I am the first to point out that correlation does not always equal causation. We can surmise that a correlated factor has a causative nature if we also see: 1) a sound rationale for why it might be occurring, 2) studies showing the mechanisms by which it occurs and 3) further studies demonstrating these effects and outcomes in vivo (in the body).

[17]

It is clear to me that people have not been ignoring the dietary guidelines for health. They have been succeeding in following them and in the process worsening their outcomes. And so it isn't that our commitment or diligence are lacking, but instead that the dietary guidelines themselves are flawed.

In my earliest days in clinical practice, I was lucky enough to work with several clients in what I termed the '200+ club'. These were people over 200 kg of bodyweight. Typically, they had been bounced around between doctors, specialists and hospital dietitians and given the same old tired advice to eat a high-carbohydrate diet, low in total and saturated fat and to continue to reduce calories until they lost weight. To maintain any weight loss they then had to continue to starve themselves to 'keep the weight off'. You can guess that this strategy was about as effective as smacking yourself in the forehead with a jandal—difficult, uncomfortable and not much fun for anyone.

Through lower-carbohydrate strategies (including ketogenic diets) we were able to achieve remarkable results: improved blood markers of health (lipids, blood glucose, and inflammatory markers), drastic improvements in weight, and most importantly improved satiety, compliance, cognition, energy and overall satisfaction. For some of these patients, it was a veritable epiphany to find strategies that were both empowering and nourishing.

[18]

And yet in spite of this success and the massive improvement in every measurable marker of good health several dietitians and doctors suggested that my interventions were dangerous and, at least, a few even went so far as to suggest that I might be putting people's lives in danger. My retort was simply: *Where is your evidence?*

I am safe in the knowledge that these people were probably given longer, happier lives because we looked outside the norm of the prevailing dietary paradigm and found a clinical intervention that worked *for them.*

CHAPTER 3

OUR FLAWED DIETARY GUIDELINES

Why demonising fat & deifying carbs isn't serving us

Dietary guidelines have not tacitly allowed a significant rise in sugar and highly refined and processed carbohydrates that have greatly increased total carbohydrate intake. They have actively condoned it.

An excessive intake of these processed and refined carbohydrate types are obvious and universally recognised risk factors for increased diabetes, obesity and metabolic dysfunction. Despite some recent positive changes (especially with respect to better guidelines for sugar intake), standard health and nutrition guidelines still typically advocate a high carbohydrate, low fat (HCLF) diet for the preservation of general health, and for the prevention or adjunctive treatment of metabolic disorders and other conditions.

Diabetes New Zealand continues to recommend a diet containing 3-4 serves of fruit per day in addition to 3-4 serves of a carbohydrate rich food (such as bread, pasta or other grain-based food) at *every meal*.[8] This provides between 180 and 240 g of carbohydrate per day (based on a standard carbohydrate serving providing 15 grams of carbohydrate)[9, 10] before even taking into account the extra carbohydrate content provided by milk and yoghurt, and fibrous vegetables, nuts and seeds. Remember that this (high-carbohydrate) recommendation is for people who have a condition that restricts their ability to dispose of carbohydrate properly!

Nutrient Reference Values (NRV) for New Zealand and Australia state that the diet should contain a minimum of 45% of its calories from carbohydrate.[11] New Zealand Heart Foundation position statements on carbohydrate (currently being updated) suggest a range of 55%-65% caloric intake should be obtained from carbohydrate, along with reducing intake of total and saturated fat.[12] These guidelines stand in contrast to the now universal recognition of the role that dysglycaemia (poor blood sugar control) has on the progression of cardiovascular diseases.[13-16]

The World Health Organisation (WHO) published dietary guidelines in 1998 suggesting a range of 55%-70% of calories should come from carbohydrate,[17] but a 2007 update suggested *that there is little evidence for the lower threshold* [my emphasis] and that this could be lowered to 50% [or less] of calories.[18]

A recommendation without evidence seems to be little more than guessing...surely?

All of these institutional recommendations would be considered moderate-to-high in carbohydrate,[19] yet there is little evidence supporting an optimal level of carbohydrate required for health. In fact, because carbohydrates are not an essential nutrient[i] (as there is no obligate requirement for carbohydrate in the diet)[20] there is little if any evidence for even a *minimum* level of carbohydrate intake—because there isn't one. That's the thing with non-essential nutrients—we don't *need* them, and so they should be considered discretionary, or as with many amino acids, considered 'conditionally essential'. In other words, they are beneficial for some people, for some purposes, but in varying amounts dependent on the needs of the individual.

The functions of the body that require carbohydrate (i.e. glycolytic energy provision for red blood cells and neurons) are provided by the creation of glucose (gluconeogenesis) from amino acids (protein) and glycerol (the 'backbone' of fats). Almost all cells can utilise lipid derived fuels such as fatty acids (via alpha- and beta-oxidation), except cells lacking mitochondria such as red blood cells. Many cell types (such as neurons and cardiac tissue) have a high affinity for the use of ketone body fuels

---

[i] 'Essential' in nutrition means that is must be consumed in the diet.

created from fat (and some amino acids) in times of carbohydrate scarcity, along with short and medium chain fatty acids.

Lower-carbohydrate diets have shown great promise for the treatment of obesity, diabetes and metabolic syndrome, neurological disorders, cancer, and have potential applications for heart disease prevention and improve some aspects of sports performance.[21, 22] In spite of this and almost without exception, they are ignored by the major dietary organisations responsible for our health and wellbeing.

CASE STUDY: NEW ZEALAND ACADEMICS TAKE ISSUE WITH THE DIETARY GUIDELINES FOR HEALTH

In 2014, submissions were called for from interested parties by the New Zealand Ministry of Health about proposed amendments to the dietary guidelines for health. The proposed guidelines involved only cosmetic changes to the existing guidelines that myself and colleagues at AUT University in Auckland, New Zealand considered to be inadequate in light of the current state of the evidence.

A working group was assembled to table a submission to the Ministry. This group consisted of Professor Grant Schofield, Dr Mikki Williden, Dr Caryn Zinn, Catherine Crofts and George Henderson (AUT), Dr

Simon Thornley (Auckland University) and myself (AUT and The Holistic Performance Institute).

In the preamble to our evaluation of the evidence Professor Schofield wrote:

"It is our contention that this [current dietary guidelines] has (partially) contributed harm to public health, especially the most vulnerable in the population. We believe this to be relevant particularly to the "demonisation" of dietary fat, the now refuted lipid hypothesis, and an emphasis on consuming large amounts of dietary carbohydrate."

It was, and remains clear to my colleagues and me that 'best-practice' guidelines have hindered rather than helped many in society, and have helped to create confusion and worsened outcomes.

THE DIETARY GUIDELINES IN QUESTION WERE:

1)   To be a healthy weight, balance your intake of food and drinks with your activity levels.

2)   Enjoy a variety of nutritious foods every day including: a) plenty of different coloured vegetables and fruit, b) a range of grains and cereals that are naturally high in fibre, c) some low fat milk products and/or calcium-fortified milk alternatives, d) some legumes, nuts, seeds, fish, eggs, lean poultry or lean red meat.

3)   Choose and prepare foods and drinks: with minimal fat, especially saturated fat; if you choose to add fat use plant-based oils and spreads; low in salt (sodium); if using salt, choose iodised salt; with little or no added sugar.

4)   Make water your first choice for drinks.

5)   Buy, prepare, cook and store food to ensure food safety.

6)   If you drink alcohol, keep your intake low. Don't drink if you are pregnant or planning to become pregnant.

We agreed with several of the proposed points for the guidelines, but also disagreed with several others for the following reasons:

OBJECTION #1: CALORIE COUNTING IS NOT FEASIBLE, NOR EFFECTIVE FOR MOST PEOPLE

"A calorie is a calorie" violates the second law of thermodynamics"[23]
A calorie is not simply a calorie.[23, 24] Simply balancing 'calories in vs. calories out' is an incomplete approach to diet as food quality and the macronutrients contained within a diet, influence outcomes (especially weight and body-composition) greatly.

Balancing intake versus output of calories is not practical for most people for any length of time. If we consider the 'auto-regulation' of calories (which we will examine later in the book) that occurs with natural, unprocessed, real-food diets, it is also unnecessary for most people, most of the time.

OBJECTION #2: WE DO NOT REQUIRE HIGH LEVELS OF GRAIN FOR HEALTH.

There is contradictory evidence about the benefits of grains and grain fibre. Although there is a role for grains in the diet for many, they are an extremely high carbohydrate-load food, and so benefits (such as the provision of vitamins such as the B vitamins [except B12] and prebiotic fibres) need to be weighed up against the potential for overloading carbohydrate.

It is important to note that many populations have lived healthily and without chronic diseases without appreciable grain intake and thus grains are not an obligate requirement in the human diet. As we shall investigate later, there is clear evidence that the historical switch to a highly grain-based diet (from a varied hunter-gatherer one) resulted in poorer health for these populations.

OBJECTION #3: THERE IS NO EVIDENCE THAT 'LOW-FAT' DAIRY IS BETTER THAN FULL-FAT.

Evidence suggests that full-fat dairy promotes better outcomes for mortality and morbidity than low-fat dairy. Full-fat dairy in combination with a diet high in fruit and vegetables exerts a protective effect against coronary artery disease (an effect not seen with low-fat dairy)[25] and colorectal cancer.[26] Contrary to the hypothesis of the authors, it was discovered that lower fat varieties of milk products (and not dairy fat) were associated with weight gain in an investigation of dairy consumption in close to 13,000 children.[27] Finally, a recent review of the literature by Kratz and colleagues concluded that the recommendation to consume low-fat dairy foods is in contrast to the observational evidence of a reduced cardiometabolic risk.[28]

OBJECTION #4: THERE IS NO COMPELLING REASON TO USE 'LEAN' MEATS OVER FATTIER CUTS

There is little to suggest that meats (and other animal tissue) higher in fat plays any significant role in mortality or morbidity.

OBJECTION #5: LITTLE EVIDENCE TO SUGGEST THAT FAT REDUCTION OR MODIFIED FAT INTAKE IMPROVES OUTCOMES.

There is little evidence suggesting that modified fat or reduced fat diets positively affect health.
For example, a Cochrane review (the 'gold standard' of systematic reviews of studies)[29] on the effect of modified or reduced fat interventions on total disease and cardiovascular disease (CVD) mortality showed no appreciable effect of the diets on either. Other reviews and meta-analyses also fail to find evidence appreciably linking reduced saturated fat intake with CVD mortality.[30, 31]

"We believe a causal effect of this dietary intervention is unlikely if there is little statistical evidence of an association between the exposure and disease."
Some studies do show a positive effect on mortality or morbidity when saturated fat replaces polyunsaturated fats (PUFAs). However these also fail to find the same

effects when monounsaturated fats or carbohydrates replace saturated fat,[32-37] so we can only determine from these studies that PUFAs (in particular the Omega 3 fats) are beneficial, not that saturated fats are harmful.

OBJECTION #6: THERE IS LITTLE EVIDENCE THAT A FAIRLY UNRESTRICTED INTAKE OF SALT IS HARMFUL TO HEALTH.

The common dietary recommendation to reduce sodium intake is based on the use of blood pressure as a marker of overall cardiovascular health. Consequently, the Adequate Intakes (AI) and the Tolerable Upper Limit (UL) for sodium set by the Institutes of Medicine of the United States National Academies[38] and endorsed by the New Zealand Ministry of Health are based on this supposed correlation.

Reducing salt intake reduces blood pressure by only between 1% and 3.5%,[39] and although this is considered statistically significant, many practitioners would suggest that this is far from *clinically significant.* To put this into context if one were to exhibit a borderline hypertension of 140/90 this would conceivably only be reduced to 135/87 in the best-case scenario by a drastic reduction in sodium intake. But when we look specifically at reductions in disease rates and deaths we find the evidence linking salt (sodium) reduction with improved outcomes is lacking and is insufficient to translate into public health recommendations. The evidence instead suggests that:

1) Reducing salt intake has no effect on population morbidity or mortality prevalence;
2) Low salt intakes negatively affect health outcomes in some population groups; and
3) Population health guidelines that are not underpinned by evidence may serve to confuse end users further, thus reducing compliance with (legitimate and scientifically robust) guidelines;
4) Reducing salt intakes further may negatively affect iodine status

Reducing sodium intake has no effect on mortality nor morbidity

A 2011 meta-analysis of RCTs of at least six months did not find evidence for reduced mortality or CVD mortality and concluded that there was no evidence available to support dietary advice to reduce salt intake. The also noted an *increase* in all-cause mortality in those with heart failure who were advised to reduce their intake.[40] The Institute of Medicine of the National Academies *Sodium Intake in Populations: Assessment of Evidence*[41] noted that:

- Reductions in sodium worsen outcomes for those with congestive heart failure.
- There are adverse health outcomes associated with sodium intake levels in ranges approximating 1,500 to 2,300 mg per day in those with diabetes, chronic kidney disease (CKD), or pre-existing CVD.
- There is no significant correlation between improved health outcomes and reductions in dietary sodium.

So the recommended (low) sodium intake amount has little benefit to normal populations and can worsen outcomes for those most at risk!

Current sodium intakes are safe

Mortality and morbidity are increased at both high and low levels of sodium intake,[43, 44] suggesting a 'U-shaped curve' of disease and disorder related to extremes of intake (either high or low). The range within which no discernible health effects are seen lies somewhere between 2,645 and 4,945 mg, or as high as 6000 mg.[43, 44]

The average intake of sodium in New Zealand is around 3900 mg per day,[45] a level well within the range that is indicated to have no appreciable effect (positive or negative) on health and so the recommendation to reduce sodium intake seems confusing and ultimately unnecessary.

Further reductions in salt intake may increase iodine deficiency

Iodised salt has played an important role in reducing iodine deficiency and goitre in New Zealand. But dietary exposure to iodine has steadily decreased since 1982,[46, 47] due mainly to the implementation of low-salt guidelines.

WHAT WE INSTEAD PROPOSED:

"THE REAL FOOD GUIDELINES"

AN ALTERNATIVE SET OF DIETARY GUIDELINES FOR NEW ZEALANDERS

1) Enjoy nutritious foods everyday including plenty of fresh vegetables and fruit.
2) Buy and prepare food from whole, unprocessed sources of dairy, nuts, seeds, eggs, meat, fish and poultry.
3) Keep sugar, added sugars, and processed foods to a minimum in all foods and drinks.
4) If you drink alcohol, keep your intake low. Don't drink if you are pregnant or planning to become pregnant.
5) Prepare, cook, and eat minimally processed traditional foods with family, friends, and your community
6) Discretionary calories (energy foods) should:
   a) Favour minimally refined grains and legumes, properly prepared, over refined or processed versions.
   b) Favour traditional oils fats and spreads over refined and processed versions.

We feel that a simpler, more pragmatic set of dietary guidelines for health that seeks to reconnect people with real food and with each other, is not only less confusing but is more effective and also based on the strongest available current evidence.

You can read the report in its entirety here:
http://www.holisticperformancenutrition.com/uploads/3/0/9/9/3099302/moh_dietary_guidelines_feedback_revised_23.4.14.pdf

CHAPTER 4

HUNTING & GATHERING

Ethnographic evidence for lower-carbohydrate diets

It is clear that humans have only eaten an appreciable amount of the very high-carbohydrate foods (in particular, grains) for a fairly short time in their overall development. For many thousands of years' humans survived as hunter-gatherers and it is only in the past several thousand (an evolutionary 'blink of the eye') that we have shifted to an agrarian existence in which grain-based foods dominate our food supply. It is even more recently that we began to eat the vast amounts of highly processed and refined (highly glycaemic loading) foods that now make up the bulk of the modern diet.

At the time of the invention and rapid uptake of agriculture around 10,000 years ago, people's height decreased and health suffered.[48] While we tend to think that having an abundant supply of food would preserve health and performance the opposite appears to have taken place.

The primary rationale for an agrarian existence is a socio-economic one, not one based on optimising health. The primary function of this food security is to ensure the resistance of the population to famine and not to ensuring the best health of individuals within that population. It allows the provision of food to a working populace and this, in turn, encourages a more rigid societal hierarchy to emerge in which poor-quality food items (staple grains) feed a working underclass.

A diet based on few staple crops provides less variety of nutrients than one based on hunted and foraged foods. This had the effect of practically malnourishing people and leaving them more susceptible to diseases that also became more prevalent due to both closer living conditions and zoomorphic infections transmitted by farm animals. While it was previously thought that the shift towards agriculture allowed an increase in population that was at least partially related to improved health, it is now generally recognised that there was a reduction in individual physical health with the abandonment of a hunter-gatherer lifestyle.

By looking at extant hunter-gatherer populations, we can see some of the best evidence for not only how humans have eaten over the course of our progression as a species but also how this affects health. Until relatively recently hunter-gatherer groups have subsisted healthily (notwithstanding mortality from infectious diseases, warfare or predation unrelated to diet) with a significant absence of metabolic disorder on a lower-carbohydrate diet.

The Inuit for example, are a population that has by necessity utilised a low-carbohydrate diet for millennia. Their diet contains a significant amount of protein (approximately 377 g of protein per day), equating to around 47% of the daily calories, with 46% coming from fat, and carbohydrate providing a mere 7% of calories.[49] Likewise, Aboriginal diets in Australia have been extensively studied. The traditional Aboriginal diet is low in carbohydrate and promoted the maintenance of lean body weights and minimised insulin resistance. When Aboriginals transition to a modern western diet that is high in carbohydrate and refined fats, the incidence of metabolic disorders, obesity and diabetes rise markedly but interestingly even a temporary reversion to a traditional hunter-gatherer lifestyle causes 'striking improvements' in carbohydrate and lipid metabolism.[50]

Hunter-gatherer populations will prioritise fatty tissue (such as bone marrow and organs) if able, to avoid spoilage and loss of nutrient dense organ meat and to provide the maximum amount of calories (and micronutrients) but perhaps most importantly to avoid the dire metabolic consequences of protein overconsumption.[51]

This is congruent with both the hunter and scavenger-dominant theories of human food acquisition, especially as both hunting and predator-confrontational scavenging are likely to have provided a large amount of the food for early humans.[52] Fresh kills by both hominids themselves and other predators would have provided organ tissue and bone marrow—both high in fat (and fat soluble vitamins), with the relatively lean tissue of wild game meats being a secondary fuel source to the fattier, and thereby more calorically and nutritionally dense tissue of organs and bone.

It should be noted, that there is considerable variation in the macronutrient content of hunter-gatherer diets. 229 hunter-gatherer diets from around the world were analysed using plant-to-animal subsistence ratios. A high variance in carbohydrate intake was found (approximately 3%-50% of daily calories).

Carbohydrate intake is inversely associated with latitude. In extremes of latitude (such as the Northern Tundra environments) higher proportions of animal derived foods, and hence, protein and fat are consumed due to the relative abundance of large game-animals. In comparison, higher carbohydrate foods such as fruits, tubers and grains are more plentiful closer to the equator. However, the authors noted that independent of the local environment the range of energy intake derived from carbohydrate in most hunter-gatherer populations is lower than the current dietary recommendations,[53] and so the recommended *minimum* amount of carbohydrate for modern humans is higher than the intakes of any of the hunter-gatherer populations studied. This begs the question: *Have we in the last 50 years discovered a better diet than the one that we evolved to eat over many millennia?*

THE ASIAN CONUNDRUM

The question invariably arises—*what about East Asian (and other) populations that eat high carbohydrate diets and that exhibit longevity and robust good health?*

One cannot answer this question without first stating unequivocally that *high carbohydrate diets are not 'bad'!* As with any other food compound or chemical, dose and exposure define the poison! And in the case of carbohydrate, there will be tolerable, and indeed a beneficial level of intake that will vary depending on someone's genetic makeup, their activity levels and a unique metabolic state, conditioned over a lifetime of eating, sleep (or lack thereof) and stress.

GENETIC TOLERANCE TO CARBOHYDRATE

From a clinician's point of view, it is clear that varying amounts of the macronutrients (protein, carbohydrates and fats) affect individuals differently, and while there are best-practice guidelines for various desired outcomes, there is a large degree of individuality between the nutritional prescriptions for individuals.

This biochemical individuality (or metabolic tolerance) has led to ideas such as *metabolic typing*—an attempt to better define what someone should eat based on a questionnaire of physical characteristics and dietary (and

[37]

other) behaviours. But there is little if any evidence to suggest that it is effective. A pilot trial of rugby players in New Zealand found that the test results did not match up with laboratory analysis of fat and carb oxidation rates.[54]

There currently is no accepted, credible way to determine the macronutrient requirements or 'tolerance' of an individual except for self-experimentation (which we will cover in our 'Step-Wise Approach to Nutrition'). There may, however, be a significant correlation between obesity and the copy number variants of a gene that codes for salivary amylase (*AMY1 CNV*),[55] the enzyme that begins the digestion of carbohydrate in the mouth. Research also suggests that *AMY1* copy number varies substantially among individuals and population groups.[56]

Populations which traditionally consume higher protein and lower starch diets have fewer copy numbers of *AMY1* compared to those from agricultural societies where starch is a prominent fuel source.[56] The *AMY1* copy number variation is likely to have evolved from nutritional pressures to facilitate the digestion of starch and may contribute to overall nutritional status.[57]

We can conclude that there is likely to be variation between ethnic groupings in their tolerance to carbohydrate and that many East Asians, by nature of these genetic differences, have a higher tolerance for carbohydrate in the diet.

COHORT EVIDENCE SUGGESTS A *LOWER-CARB, HIGH-CARB DIET* PROMOTES BETTER OUTCOMES IN A HIGH-CARB CONSUMING, EAST ASIAN POPULATION

There is evidence to suggest that a lower-carb variant of a high-carb diet is still superior to an arbitrarily high diet in a carb-tolerant East Asian population. In a study of over 10,000 Japanese conducted over 29 years, those consuming lower carbohydrate amounts had slightly improved mortality rates (which were statistically significant for women).[58]

It is clear that there is considerable variation in tolerance to carbohydrate (and by extension the other macronutrients) between individuals and that this has a genetic and conditioned foundation. It is unwise to suggest that because a particular diet is good for one population that it is inherently good for the rest. It is also clear that some populations do extremely well on a high carbohydrate diet and that I consider it to be wholly appropriate for them. But even in these cases, there is likely to be a point at which the intake of any non-essential nutrient (i.e. carbohydrate) will reach a 'tipping-point' of safety and after this, higher intakes are likely to lead to progressively increasing health risks. Critics may argue that the same will occur with any of the macronutrients—and I whole heartedly agree! The question that needs to be asked though (and I suggest that we have already answered it) is *'Are our current blanket recommendations in contrast to what is most evolutionarily appropriate for the human animal?'*

CHAPTER 5

STARVING ON A FULL STOMACH

Micronutrient insufficiency & metabolic
starvation

It seems counter-intuitive to think that in the modern world, in which we eat more than ever before and have an environment of surplus rather than scarcity that we could be starving. But in spite of a surplus of calories, we may not, in fact, be getting all that we need from the modern diet to truly thrive.

STARVING FOR NUTRIENT DENSITY

Vitamins and minerals act as co-factors for literally thousands of chemical reactions throughout the body— from facilitating the breakdown of foods into energy, through to cellular reproduction, expression of genes and much more. Suffice it to say that without enough of the 'little guys' of nutrition, nothing much can occur in the body. I like to think of the micronutrients (vitamins and minerals) being like the spark plugs in a car. They don't provide the fuel directly but allow its efficient use.

United States Department of Agriculture (USDA) data shows that some fresh produce (vegetables, fruits berries) only provide around half the amounts of some vitamins and minerals that they did in the 1950s.[59] To get the same amounts of nutrients, we need to eat twice the amount of some veggies and other 'nutrient dense' foods than we did 50 or so years ago.

Makes you wonder whether '5+ a day' is going to cut it for you?

Estimates from the New Zealand Ministry of Health 'NZ Adult Nutrition Survey' of 2008/2009 suggest that many New Zealanders are not getting the recommended amounts of many of the vitamins and minerals from their diets.[60]

Some of the key findings included:

- Around 20% of people fail to get sufficient vitamins A, B1 and B6.
- 8% of people fail to get sufficient B12.
- Nearly 10% of women don't get enough iron.
- Around 25% of people don't consume enough zinc. Interestingly nearly 40% of males do not get adequate zinc from their diet.
- 45% of people don't get enough Selenium (a mineral lacking in New Zealand soils).

So we know that some of the food we eat, even if we are trying to eat a 'good' diet, may be less nutritious than it once was and further, that we need to eat more nutrient-dense foods to supply what we require to thrive. We simply do not eat enough of these nutrient-dense foods to supply what we require day-to-day from the food we currently eat.

STARVING FOR FUEL…

In spite of ample calories, we are still 'functionally starving'.

A 'calorie is a calorie' has been found to be inadequate,[23] and many of our models of fuel utilisation and substrate storage are outdated.

Altered satiety signals are both a causative factor and result from metabolic disorder and obesity.[61-63] When we have a metabolic disorder or are obese, we have distorted satiety signals along with a reduced ability to adequately digest and assimilate some nutrients, along with a reduced ability to store and use fuels optimally. Thus, even if eating more than we require, we can still find ourselves lacking in readily available fuel.

This line of thinking provides a significant challenge as we have typically considered it impossible to 'starve' if we are getting bigger—because most surely in a state of caloric surplus we should have enough fuel. But this is not necessarily true. When we have a predisposition to storing fat, we may not have sufficient fuel stored within tissue because we are unable to store efficiently. Our rates of fat utilisation can be markedly reduced, and we, therefore, have greater difficulty 'freeing' up fuel from fat-storage (adipose tissue) due to distortions in our enzymatic ability to release fat from cells and to uptake triglycerides (fats) into muscle and other cells for use. We are also at risk of becoming more and more insulin resistant—with a reduced ability to dispose of glucose, despite having developed a preference for using glucose (sugar) as fuel!

The good news is that changes in the macronutrient composition of what we eat (i.e. the relative amounts of fat vs. carbohydrate vs. protein) can positively affect weight, body-composition and cardiometabolic outcomes.

HIGH PROTEIN, LOW CARBOHYDRATE DIETS

Due to simple calorie displacement, low-carbohydrate diets require an increase in one or both of the other macronutrients (protein or fat) to fulfil caloric requirements, although calorie restricted lower-carbohydrate diets may simply reduce carbohydrate and thereby increase the relative proportions of fat and protein. High-protein, low-carbohydrate (HPLC) diets enhance weight-loss with greater loss of body-fat and reduced loss of lean body mass due to factors including increased satiety, increased thermogenesis, muscle sparing and improved glycaemic (blood sugar) control.[64]

High-protein, low-carbohydrate diets have been studied for weight-loss and body composition with superior results demonstrated versus high-carbohydrate diets.

Layman and colleagues compared two diets with similar fat content (~50 g), one containing 68 g protein and the other 125 g (with the balance in both cases from carbohydrate). Participants in the higher protein group lost significantly more fat, retained more lean tissue, and reduced triacylglycerol (TAG) and increased satiety more than the lower protein group.[65]

Piatti and colleaguesinvestigated the effects of two hypocaloric diets (800 kcal) in normal, glucose tolerant women, one containing 45% protein (35% carbohydrate [CHO] and 20% fat) and one containing 20% protein (60% CHO, 20% fat). Similar weight loss occurred in both groups, but retention of fat-free mass (muscle) was only seen in the higher protein diet.[66]

Similarly, in obese and hyperinsulinaemic women a higher protein intake (27% vs. 16%) and similar fat intakes encouraged similar weight and fat loss with retention of lean mass only observed in the higher protein group, along with reduced TAG and improved glycaemic control versus the lower-protein, higher-carbohydrate group.[67]

Noakes and others have demonstrated that there may be further nutritional benefits resulting from higher protein diets—with a greater fat loss in the obese, reduced TAG and improved B12 status compared to higher carbohydrate diets.[68] In a comparison of a high-protein (30%) versus high-carbohydrate (55%) isocaloric diet (n=11), individuals on a high protein diet lost more fat with no difference observed between fat-free mass between groups.[69]

The positive effects of higher protein intake on body-composition can be explained due to several factors, including increased satiety and thermogenesis when compared to equivalent amounts of either carbohydrates or fat.[70] Increased energy expenditure (EE) results from the formation of additional glucose from amino acids (and other substrates such as lactate and glycerol).[71] There is also a higher thermic effect of feeding (TEF) (using more calories) from protein ingestion as compared to either carbohydrate or fat.[72-74] Increased caloric expenditure resulting from protein intake is not explained solely by the metabolic demands of increased gluconeogenesis and may also be accounted for by increased protein accretion in tissue, which requires greater energy expenditure than for storage of fat within adipose tissue.[75] There is a large amount of both lay and scientific literature showing increased protein accretion and retention with higher protein intakes.

However, only moderate increases in protein and minor reductions in carbohydrate have not been shown to provide increased resting energy expenditure (REE) nor promote appreciably greater loss of body-fat.[76] It is likely that more severe carbohydrate restriction or a much greater protein intake are the variables that promote the greatest reductions in body-fat, and in the case of high protein intakes, have the greatest effect on diet induced energy expenditure.

Higher protein intake is also considered to be more satiating than the carbohydrate it is displacing. A 2004 review by Halton and Hu found there to be convincing evidence that a higher protein intake increases thermogenesis and satiety compared to diets of a lower protein content.[77]

HPLC diets are often misrepresented as ketogenic diets. If there is either insufficient total fat intake or insufficient Medium Chain Triglyceride (MCT) intake to either qualify as a 'classic' or MCT ketogenic diet respectively, there is unlikely to be the rise in blood ketone levels (ketonaemia) to constitute a 'functional' or 'nutritional' ketosis. An extremely high level of protein in the diet is also likely to be glucogenic (in other words the excess amino acids are converted into glucose) and thus anti-ketogenic.

Where a higher protein diet (for example at ~ 30% of calories) has extremely low carbohydrate (and thereby sufficient fat intake), it is likely to provide sufficient ketone production to be ketogenic. Johnstone and colleagues demonstrated that an ad-libitum diet of this type (low-carb, high-protein ketogenic diet) offers greater satiety and increased weight-loss over a moderate carbohydrate, high protein diet, due probably to a greater auto-restriction of calories in the ketogenic diet group.[78]

Low Carbohydrate, High Fat (LCHF) diets

Low carbohydrate, high fat diets (often with low-to-moderate protein) likewise have demonstrated sufficient evidence to be considered a therapeutic option for the primary and adjunctive treatment of fatty liver disease[79]; type 1 diabetes[80]; type 2 diabetes[81]; cancer[82]; and cognitive impairment.[83]

LCHF diets are likely to be superior to low-fat diets for improving several markers of cardiovascular health with the possible exception of low-density lipoprotein (LDL).[84-86] LDL cholesterol is used as a proxy for cardiovascular health and is commonly known as 'bad cholesterol'. In fact, it's a cholesterol 'carrier' protein which transports vital cholesterol to peripheral tissue where it provides a component of cell membranes and is used to create the steroid hormones. High-density lipoprotein (HDL), known as 'good cholesterol' brings cholesterol back to to liver for conversion and eventual excretion as bile. It's important to have a healthy balance of these cholesterol carriers and triglycerides (fats) in the blood.

HDL-to-total cholesterol ratio appears to relate more closely to improved cardiovascular mortality than LDL levels, and this ratio is more favourably impacted by an LCHF diet in comparison to a higher carbohydrate diet.[87] Beneficial lipid sub-fractions (including large particle LDL) are also increased favourably with an LCHF diet.[88] (See Appendix A 'Cholesterol')

LCHF diets could provide the 'metabolic advantage' of greater retention of lean mass, with greater fat-loss when compared to higher carbohydrate diets providing the same amount of calories. This effect has been demonstrated in studies since the 1960s.[89] A metabolic advantage does not contravene the laws of energy conservation (the first law of thermodynamics) as there are inefficiencies and efficiencies within the human body's systems based on the macronutrients we eat and the thermic effect of these can provide a net calorie loss.[23, 24] Other factors such as the effect on protein synthesis resulting from higher levels of protein and essential amino acids (EAAs)[90, 91] such as leucine (the 'signalling' amino acid for protein synthesis)[92] may encourage increased protein synthesis[93, 94] which in itself creates increased caloric expenditure. Anti-catabolic effects of higher fat intakes and the resultant 'fat-adaptation' which reduces the need for tissue breakdown to facilitate gluconeogenesis may also encourage increased fat-loss. These and other factors are likely to influence the metabolic and anthropometric advantages provided by HPLC and LCHF diets.

Short term studies suggest that carbohydrate restriction—irrespective of what is substituted, has the greatest effect on weight-loss. For example, a 2005 randomised controlled trial by Luscombe-Marsh et al. compared a low carbohydrate high protein diet to a low carbohydrate, high fat (standard protein) diet—both yielding similar results for weight loss with little difference in other parameters (bone turnover, inflammation and calcium excretion).[95]

Lower-carbohydrate and higher-fat diets (not 'LCHF' per se) have demonstrated improved post-prandial glycaemic responses and reduced insulin when compared to higher-protein, isocaloric diets.[96]

CHAPTER 6

METABOLIC EFFICIENCY

Finding your level of carb-tolerance with Holistic
Performance Nutrition

From a clinicians point of view it is clear that differing amounts of the macronutrients (protein, carbohydrates and fats) affect individuals differently, and while there are best-practice guidelines for various desired outcomes, there is a large degree of individuality between the prescription for individuals.

This variability has been termed by practitioners; *biochemical individuality* or *metabolic typing*, however, there is, at this point in time, no accepted way to determine more finely the macronutrient requirements or 'tolerance' of an individual, except in those cases where a specific diet benefits a disease or disorder (such as a ketogenic diet for epilepsy).

In clinical practice carbohydrate intake is often adjusted the most, because of its non-essentiality.[20] Because carbohydrate is not essential, and yet can be extremely beneficial but in widely differing amounts for individuals, we need to be able to evaluate better what those differences may be.

Due to its nature as an almost exclusively fuel-providing substrate it is self-evident that carbohydrate intake rests upon two major factors:

1) The activity level of the individual (latent activity from habits and nervous and 'constitutional' behaviours, work-type, and exercise intensity, frequency and volume)
2) The metabolic tolerance to carbohydrate—which is likely to be dependent on genetic predisposition, and to exercise/activity and to dietary and medical history, especially where these factors may contribute to a tendency towards insulin resistance.

The difficult part for anyone is to try to figure out their unique tolerance to the macronutrients. One could begin by counting calories and macronutrients and adjusting these to attempt to find an optimal range of intake, but this is often tedious, ultimately unsustainable, and is for most people unnecessary (as we shall see in the following pages). On the other hand, a 'step-wise' restriction of certain food types can be enormously helpful in finding a level of carb intake that meets your metabolic tolerance and activity based requirements.

STEP 1. NATURAL, WHOLE & UNPROCESSED

People over-complicate nutrition and rush into using diets with extreme restrictions or excessive supplementation, when minor changes, applied with consistency will give greater results.

Small and consistent changes are easy to implement and integrate into your daily routine and can more easily become positive habits that 'stick'. Conversely doing more than what is necessary to achieve your goal is a wasted effort and can be counterproductive in the long-term—for example if you unnecessarily restrict a food type that you can eat without ill-effect.

Eat a diet that contains 80% Natural, Whole and Unprocessed Foods (ad libitum)

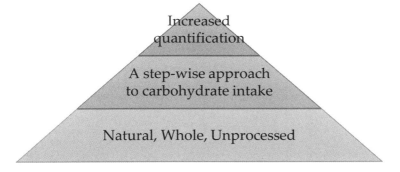

Figure 3. A Hierarchy of Priorities for Nutrition. By the author.

It is likely that diets based almost entirely around natural, unprocessed foodstuffs provide a degree of 'metabolic advantage' like that seen in studies on low-carbohydrate diets, yet without the absolute necessity of intentionally restricting carbohydrate. While critics may point to a relative paucity of research on diets that emphasise whole, unprocessed foodstuffs (such as 'The Paleo Diet'), there is emerging and compelling evidence for the beneficial effects of real-food diets. Paleo, while often derided by orthodox dieticians and medical practitioners, has a growing body of evidence which suggests compelling benefits.

- Satiety
  A Paleo meal may provide greater satiety than a standard meal based on 'best-practice' dietary guidelines,[97] best-practice diabetic meal plan,[98] and the Mediterranean Diet.[99]

- Cardiometabolic Risk Factors
  Paleo diets reduce cholesterol, LDL cholesterol, triglycerides, insulin and blood pressure.[100, 101] A randomised controlled trial featuring nine men and 25 women found that a Paleo diet resulted in lower blood pressure, cholesterol, triglycerides and higher HDL cholesterol than the reference diet over two weeks. No differences were noted for intestinal permeability ('leaky gut'), inflammation or salivary cortisol (a marker of stress). A randomised cross-over trial featuring ten men and three women demonstrated that Paleo diets have a lower glycaemic index and are lower in total energy compared to a diabetic diet. The Paleo diet resulted in lower HbA1c (a measure of average blood sugar levels), triglycerides, blood pressure and higher HDL cholesterol.

- Fat Loss

  In a two year randomised controlled trial, post-menopausal women lost more fat at six months and had lower triglycerides at six and 24 months.[102] Ten healthy post-menopausal women ate *ad libitum* (eat as much as you want) on a Paleo diet for five weeks. Average calorie intake was reduced by 25%, and average weight loss was 4.5 kg along with reduced waist and hip circumference, blood pressure, fasting glucose, cholesterol, triglycerides and LDL cholesterol (fat in the liver – a marker for metabolic disorder was also decreased).[103]

Diets that emphasise REAL, WHOLE food, are also likely to:

- Provide increased amounts of a complex array of both primary and secondary nutrients
- Provide prebiotic, gut-supporting fibres and resistant starches without increasing glycaemic load in a disproportionate manner
- Reduced glycaemic load in total
- Preserve fat quality
- Provide ample amounts of all macro- and micro-nutrients
- Aid auto-regulation of calories

The absolute priority for any change in diet should be to focus initially on the *quality* of food eaten, not just *quantities*. Many people will find that simply applying a greater focus to eating a diet that is based almost exclusively on natural, unprocessed foods will not need to be any more restrictive or prescriptive.

ARE 'PALEO' STYLE DIETS SAFE?

The premise of the paleo diet is that genetically we haven't changed much since the time of the earliest humans. It has been said that *"From a genetic standpoint, humans living today are Stone Age hunter-gatherers displaced through time to a world that differs from that for which our genetic constitution was selected"*.[104]

Hunter-gatherer populations such as the Inuit, Australian Aboriginals, Hadza and others have until recent times lived relatively healthily and with a significant absence of the metabolic disorders of obesity and diabetes that plague the modern, western world.[49, 50, 105, 106]

The 'modern' Paleo diet seeks to emulate these traditional hunter-gatherer diets by eliminating foods that are abundant in the modern diet but that were not present (in large amounts) in the diets of most hunter-gatherers. There are many variations on the Paleo theme and most people now follow some iteration of Paleo that could differ from the original template. For example, many now would classify their diet as 'Primal', a style of nutrition in itself quite diverse but typically being similar to Paleo but with the addition of some dairy and occasionally sprouted legumes and even occasional grains. The following table describes Paleo food choices.

[56]

Eat	Avoid
Free range, organic meat, eggs, fish	Factory farmed meats, battery eggs
Nuts and seeds	
Fibrous vegetables	
Root vegetables (sweet potato, yams, etc.)	Grains and legumes
Berries and fruit	
Virgin nut and fruit oils (olive, macadamia, coconut)	Seed oils, dairy

Table 1. Paleo food guide. By the author.

DID PALEOLITHIC MAN *REALLY* EAT LIKE THAT?

Critics of the Paleo diet point to the lack of consistency in hunter-gatherer diets. In other words, there is no 'one true' hunter-gatherer diet. For example, analysis of 229 hunter-gatherer diets from around the world found a high variance in carbohydrate intake (approximately 3%-50% of daily calories). However, the authors noted that carbohydrate intake in almost all hunter-gatherer populations is lower than that currently recommended for health,[53] and it's fair to say that all hunter gatherer populations have an absence of refined and processed foods! It's also interesting to note that many critics of real-food based diets like Paleo are advocates for the Mediterranean Diet, and yet there is no 'one' Mediterranean Diet either. It is more important to look at either diet (because they are both great!) not as rigid prescriptions of certain foods for all people, but instead a compendium of available foods from which to choose.

[57]

IS PALEO OK FOR WOMEN?

The few trials that have been performed on the Paleo diet and those including women specifically overwhelmingly show benefits, with no adverse effects reported.

Much of the criticism of Paleo diets for women come from the assumption that a Paleo diet is low in carbohydrate and that this might negatively affect thyroid status or cause other hormone imbalances. However, the Paleo diet isn't by nature low in carbohydrates as it can (depending on how it's applied) include appreciable carbohydrate from sweet potato, yams, vegetables, berries and some fruit, which would be more than adequate for most women.

PALEO AND HORMONES

There is no good reason to think that a Paleo diet would negatively affect hormone levels. However, a *severely carb-restricted* Paleo diet can affect hormone levels in *some* women. Carbohydrate restriction can increase cortisol levels (one of our major stress hormones), although this hasn't been noted in the existing work on the Paleo diet, and reduce levels of the sex hormones (especially testosterone). This cortisol to free testosterone ratio is a key marker of fatigue syndromes. It is important to note that much of these distortions occur in the transition phase to a lower carbohydrate diet, but typically do not last if one becomes sufficiently 'fat adapted'.

MEAL TIMING

Meal timing and frequency is certainly not as important as was once thought. Whereas we have been told that we need to drip-feed nutrients into the system, we now know that more infrequent feedings are completely appropriate for many people.

This makes complete sense if we think about the physiology of the human organism. It is extremely well adapted to go through periods of fasting and periods of feeding. When we are active during the day, we are 'sympathetic nervous system (SNS) dominant'. This is our so-called 'fight or flight' response. In this state, we release higher levels of the stress hormones, especially epinephrine and norepinephrine. These allow greater cognition (to a point) and help the body to free glucose for immediate use as fuel. The body also seeks to prioritise blood supply to working muscles and reduces blood flow to the gastrointestinal tract and visceral organs and also closes gastric sphincters (valves) and reduces motility (movement) through the bowel. All these factors of the stress-response reduce our ability to utilise food effectively during times of activity and so it makes sense to simply be active and to wait to eat until we get a chance (or more so in the modern world, make the time!) to eat.

Our parasympathetic nervous system (when in dominance) is known conversely as the 'rest and digest' system. In this state we relax, gastric enzymes and hydrochloric acid are produced in greater amounts and movement of food through the bowel is prioritised.

For this reason, when people ask what they should eat when 'on the run' I tell them: "Don't eat on the run!" A better strategy is to allow yourself to be active, but then when you make a time to stop, actually stop, and prepare a wholesome meal (or have one ready to go) and sit down, relax, eat it and enjoy!

The take home message for frequency is a simple one. If you are eating natural, whole foods, you should eat when you are hungry, until you are full and then eat again when hungry again! If you occasionally miss a meal don't stress about it at all.

Some people benefit from increased feeding frequency (many athletes and bodybuilders for example), but we will explore that later in the sections on quantification.

INTERMITTENT FASTING

Many years ago I was working with Islamic clients. They wondered (as did I) about the effects of Ramadan fasting on health. Interested in this I searched the available literature to see what effects if any fasting had on health and performance. I was surprised to find that what little evidence there was at the time suggested no negative effects on health and this critical piece of information shook the 'frequent eating' dogma to its core. Since then I have used fasting protocols for a variety of reasons (some mental, emotional and spiritual). Fasting isn't for everyone, and I wouldn't say that it's essential, but knowing that it exerts some benefits provides another reason not to be overly fastidious about having to eat 'by-the-clock'.

There are now hundreds of papers on intermittent fasting. Reviews of these papers suggest that intermittent fasting results in weight-loss and improved cardiometabolic risk factors including improved blood glucose profiles, insulin, cholesterol profiles and inflammatory markers.[107, 108] Experience from Ramadan studies on athletes also suggests that physical fitness is not negatively affected, and athletes who maintain an appropriate calorie (fuel) intake, hydration and preserve sleep length, don't suffer a reduction in performance doing this type of fast.[109, 110]

WHAT ABOUT ALCOHOL?

Systematic reviews of the scientific evidence suggest that a low level of alcohol intake (1-2 drinks per day) is associated with a reduced risk of Alzheimer's Disease and dementia,[111] diabetes,[112, 113] reduced HbA1C,[114] reduced risk for Ischaemic Heart Disease (IHD),[115, 116] and multiple cardiac outcomes,[117] improved cardiac markers,[118] reduced risk for nasopharyngeal carcinoma,[119] and a 10% reduction in total mortality risk,[120] and is not associated with kidney function decline[121] nor weight gain.[122] Evidence for a protective effect of low to moderate drinking on stroke occurrence is lacking[123] although light alcohol use appears associated with reduced occurrence of ischaemic stroke.[124]

A 2013 systematic review while finding (unsurprisingly) that moderate to heavy consumption of alcohol increases the risk of developing cancer of the oral cavity and pharynx, oesophagus, stomach, larynx, colorectum, central nervous system, pancreas, breast and prostate, failed to find any association between alcohol consumption and an increased risk of cancers of the lung, bladder, endometrium and ovary. It was also observed that alcohol consumption is inversely related to the occurrence of thyroid cancer.[125] Other reviews did not find any meaningful association between alcohol consumption and cancer of the ovary[126] or glioma.[127]

Colorectal adenoma is increased at all levels of alcohol consumption[128] and oesophageal, and liver cancers are increased even with moderate (approx. 2.5 drinks per day) alcohol use.[129]

WHAT DOES THIS MEAN?

The 'nadir' or dose at which total mortality is reduced most lies somewhere between seven and 12 drinks per week for men and under three drinks per week for women.[130]

It is clear that heavy drinking is detrimental socially, puts one at much greater risk of accident and violence, and increases total mortality risk along with individual risk for nearly every condition that has been studied. Current research also conclusively shows that any amount of 'binge' drinking is negative, and reverses any benefits from light alcohol use. There are also inherent risks for addiction and abuse arising from otherwise healthy use, and so the recommendation that if you don't currently drink there is no good reason to start, is a common-sense one. On the other hand, if you do drink it is prudent to keep your intake down to under seven drinks per week, with no more than two drinks per day and 'alcohol-free' days each and every week.

If you currently drink, limit your intake by only buying enough for the week. For example, I drink beer and buy no more than a dozen beers at the beginning of the week. If I finish them, that's it, no more for that week. If I don't, I roll them over to the following week *and don't restock until they are gone.* I also drink light beer as this further limits my intake to that 'nadir' amount of 7-12 drinks per week. If you drink wine buying only one bottle of wine per week is a great start.

Note: Alcohol can be problematic for weight-loss. It is not necessarily so, especially if you are drinking within these moderate, healthy limits, but if you are struggling to lose weight reducing or eliminating alcohol for a time can be a great experiment to see what works best for you.

COFFEE – TO IMBIBE OR NOT?

Coffee is frequently singled out as a 'thou shalt not' by practitioners. The evidence for this is lacking though.

Systematic reviews suggest a dose-dependent correlation between coffee intake and reduced rates of diabetes with the greatest effects seen in those consuming the highest amounts of coffee (greater than six cups per day).[131-133] For every additional cup consumed, there is an approximately 7% reduction in diabetes risk and benefits are also seen from tea and decaffeinated coffee.[134]

Coffee does increase blood pressure (BP) acutely (although these studies use high amounts in the range of 200-300 mg, approximately 2-3 cups of coffee) and this has led clinicians to urge caution with coffee intake due to a perceived risk of cardiovascular disease (CVD). But there appears to be no correlation between long-term, habitual use of coffee with cardiovascular disease or chronic high blood pressure.[135, 136] Low intakes may even be more likely to increase blood pressure with 1-3 cups demonstrating an effect on BP and 3-5 cups showing no long-term effect.[137] Likewise low intakes have been demonstrated to increase CVD risk slightly (less than three cups per day) with 3-5 cups per day associated with reduced CVD.[138]

In chronic liver disease, patients who consume coffee have a decreased risk of progression to cirrhosis, a lowered mortality rate, and in chronic hepatitis C patient coffee was associated with improved responses to antiviral therapy. Moreover, coffee consumption is inversely related to the severity of steatohepatitis (fatty liver) in those with pre-existing non-alcoholic fatty liver disease (NAFLD). It is therefore recommended that those with liver disease should be encouraged to drink coffee daily.[139] Gallstone risk is also reduced with higher coffee intakes, with the highest consumption (around six cups or more) associated with the lowest risk.[140]

Fracture risk rises in a dose dependent manner in women but not with men. There is little difference in fracture risk around two coffees per day.[141]

There does not appear to be any link between coffee consumption and gastric cancer,[142] breast cancer[143] or colorectal cancer, although there may be a small positive effect seen in women coffee drinkers.[144] There may also be a minor increase in urinary tract cancer associated with coffee drinking[145] and cancer of the larynx also rises in a dose-dependent manner.[146]

Coffee may also offer some mild protective effect against cognitive decline, dementia[147] and depression.[148]

WHAT DOES IT ALL MEAN?!

A systematic review of seventeen studies including over one million participants and 131,212 death events was conducted by Yimin Zhao and colleagues in May 2015. The review and meta-analysis determined a 'U-shaped dose–response relationship' between coffee intake and all-cause mortality. Mortality was reduced at all levels of coffee intake with the greatest effects seen at 3-5 cups.[149]

RECOMMENDATIONS

We must conclude, based on the evidence, that coffee is safe and moreover offers significant benefits to health. The reason for the benefits is likely to be multifactorial and include the effects of caffeine itself and also the range of antioxidant chemicals found in coffee. The 'nadir' or optimal health intake appears to be around 3-5 cups of coffee per day. However, this is individual dependent. As with alcohol if you do not drink coffee there is probably no good reason to start, but likewise, if you do drink coffee without any negative side effects there is absolutely no reason to stop (according to the evidence), and your daily cups/s of Joe could even be improving your health!

If you experience disrupted sleep, you may want to perform a 'self-experiment' and reduce your intake. It is always prudent to reduce or eliminate caffeine containing drinks later in the day, and a good rule-of-thumb is to have no more than 3-5 cups of coffee, with the last no later than 12-2 pm. The 'take-home' rule here is to listen to your body. If coffee disturbs your sleep, reduces your concentration ability, causes you to feel excessively fatigued during exercise; if you 'crash' after caffeine or it upsets your digestive system, then reduce or eliminate it and see how you feel. In short—look at the evidence, but be sensible and apply your n=1[i] filter!

---

[i] n=1 refers to an experiment of one person. Commonly used to describe a self-experiment.

TAKING BREAKS

Any discussion around any drug such as alcohol and coffee is fraught with challenge and confrontation. People have their biases and will 'cherry-pick' research and opinion pieces to support that decision. For this reason, I have limited my exploration of these topics to systematic reviews and meta-analyses of the evidence, so as to utilise the greatest volume of data to come to these conclusions. However, while I have tried to determine general guidelines for most people, these are a starting point only, and anyone should determine their tolerance for any substance. I can't stress highly enough that if something is not working well for you, *do not continue using it just because it is 'healthy' for someone else!*

Any substance that has psychoactive properties, or, in fact, any substance that elicits any biochemical response (even if that is a psychosocial one such as enjoyment or ritualised relaxation) has the potential to become a learned or 'patterned' response. This sitaution is similar to, but not the same as addiction. With addiction, we are typically speaking of something more serious and pathological (i.e. causing harm). Patterned and behavioural conditioning (i.e. drinking coffee every morning) is not a negative thing per se. However, it can be. An interesting exercise to recognise your patterns of behaviour is to take breaks periodically to become more mindful of the way that you respond to food, to alcohol, to coffee or other things that you rely on regularly. This enhanced mindfulness is one of the most important benefits of fasting. I fast relatively regularly, and one of the benefits is to help me to become more mindful of (true) hunger, patterned eating behaviours and those times when I am eating for a reason other than hunger (such as 'emotional eating'). I also regularly take breaks from both alcohol and coffee for the same reason. Each year I do a fairly strict variation of a traditional mystics 'Lenten' fast which involves abstinence from alcohol, coffee, sugar, meat, eggs and dairy. My reasons are predominantly spiritual for this, but the benefits for mind and body are compelling too. Releasing attachment to one's patterns is an extraordinary exercise in mindfulness and an interesting observation of the human condition. By occasionally taking breaks from the things that we habitually consume we can see just how attached we have become to them and we can also observe any potential negative effects that we previously hadn't realised. This can give us insight into foods or substances that we thought were serving us, but, in fact, weren't. In addition, taking breaks from certain things forces us to try alternatives. For example, when fasting and abstaining from meat one of the enormous benefits is to reconnect to eating more vegetables, and a greater variety of them.

If you eat meat, that's all good! (So do I) but how about taking a break for a week or two?

If you drink (lightly) that's also fine, but have you tried going without for a few weeks or a month?

If you need coffee to wake up in the morning, it might be a good idea not to have it for even a few days and try to 'get going' without the stimulant?

Change is very often a positive thing. Try taking some breaks from your dietary patterns and recognise the way your mind and body respond.

Are you getting the results you desire? If so, stick with your natural, whole, unprocessed approach to eating!
If not – move on to level 2: A Step-Wise Approach to Carb Restriction.

CHAPTER 7

FINDING *YOUR* CARB-APPROPRIATE DIET

A step-wise approach to carbohydrate restriction

Many people will experience improved health and metabolic function and begin to normalise weight and fat levels simply by eating a natural, whole-foods based, nutrient-dense diet but some may require further modifications to the diet.

You might need to restrict carbohydrate further if:

- You are metabolically disordered
- You have diabetes (type 1 or 2)
- You are genetically most suited to a lower-carbohydrate intake

An optimal carbohydrate dose (like any other nutrient) is likely to fall somewhere on a 'bell-shaped curve'. In other words, some people respond best to extremely low or high carbohydrate diets, with the vast majority falling into a range that is somewhere between these extremes.

It is likely that the average optimal range for carbohydrate for most people is lower than what the current dietary guidelines tell us for several reasons. 1) Recommendations for carbohydrate intake have consistently fallen (from 65%+ 20 years ago to around 45%+ now), 2) anthropological evidence supports lower carbohydrate intakes, and 3) carbohydrates are not an essential nutrient.

The outdated (high-carb) recommendations also don't allow for optimal intake amounts of either protein or fat for performance for most people.

If we consider the 'old-style' recommendation to eat over 65% of calories from carbohydrate, this only leaves 35% in total from both protein and fat combined.

Many experts consider an intake of at least 30% of calories from fat is necessary to ensure appropriate hormonal health (and performance).[150] If we take an example of an average, 75 kg male requiring 2200 calories this would equate to:

	65% carbohydrate	55%	45%	35%	25%
CHO (g)	357	303	248	193	138
PRO (g)	29	83	137	193	248
FAT (g)	73	73	73	73	73

Table 2. Protein amounts versus carbohydrate and fat at varying recommended intake levels. By the author.

SUGGESTED PROTEIN INTAKE PER DAY

Recommended Daily Allowance (RDA): 60 g

International Society of Sports Nutrition (ISSN) Guidelines for Performance: 105-165 g

Upper threshold demonstrated to support anthropometry: approx. 205 g

This table demonstrates that with a suggested *minimum* level of fat for performance retention higher intakes of carbohydrate do not allow sufficient protein for optimal performance. Likewise, if we were to perform similar calculations, but instead preserve optimal protein intake for performance, our fat intake would then be insufficient if consuming an extremely high carbohydrate intake.

There are obviously more ways that someone could consume their calories than those illustrated above (for example a lower-carb, *higher-fat* diet).

This table does demonstrate though that if consuming the recommended amount of fat to support hormonal health and athletic performance, and RDA and ISSN-recommended levels of protein, current recommended level of carbohydrate intake cannot be supported in the diets of most normal a*nd athletic* people.

Some people will undoubtedly benefit from higher carbohydrate recommendations. However, our clinical experience would suggest that these people are in the minority.

STRATEGY: A GRADUAL RESTRICTION OF HIGHER-CARBOHYDRATE FOODS

WHY RESTRICTION?

- Abstinence is often easier than moderation
- Allows for a simple method of elimination diet (for allergies and intolerances)
- Allows for this elimination in an easily integrated fashion and reduces potential metabolic or digestive disruptors.

ABSTINENCE IS EASIER THAN MODERATION

There is a lack of research on the effects of moderation vs. abstinence on diet outcomes. However clinical experience suggests that it is a simpler 'mind-set' for people to think of one, clear elimination strategy at a time (in which they completely avoid one particular food), rather than having to quantify *and then* reduce food types or reduce certain macronutrients and count calories.

Steps along the 'step-wise' approach serve to reduce the total glycaemic load in the diet and because lower-carb diets have demonstrated greater satiety, improved compliance and auto-regulation they allow an easier road to fat-loss than having to practically starve yourself.

BENEFITS FOR ELUCIDATING ALLERGIES AND INTOLERANCES

Elimination diets are a real-life test of intolerances to foods. In fact, many medical texts prioritise this type of elimination testing as one of the few ways to credibly determine intolerances. This is not the primary purpose of the step-wise approach, but if when following a gradual restriction of carbohydrate, you notice reduced symptoms of food intolerance (i.e., improved energy and wellbeing, reduced gastro-intestinal symptoms, improved cognitive performance and reduced skin conditions and nasal congestion), you can better identify food types to which you are intolerant.

A STEP-WISE APPROACH TO MACRONUTRIENT MANIPULATION

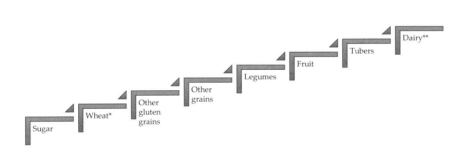

Figure 4. A step-wise approach to Carb-Appropriate nutrition.

*WHEAT AND GLUTEN

Wheat (and specifically gluten) is not the 'bogey-man' that many have made it out to be. The original research suggesting that many people have a non-coeliac gluten sensitivity was subsequently found to be at least partially inaccurate. However, some people that are not coeliac may still suffer adverse responses to wheat. It is a common allergen, and foods made from wheat flour (bread, pastries, cookies, etc.) are high-carb foods, that if avoided often result in a reduction in total carbohydrate intake that aids fat-loss.

Sequentially Avoid						
Sugar	Wheat	Gluten Grains	Other Grains	Legumes	Fruits	Tubers
Obvious sugar containing foods Honey Maple Syrup Fruit juice Soft drinks	Including breads, pasta, and savoury cookies, muesli and granola	Barley, rye or (if intolerant) oats	Such as quinoa, millet, amaranth	Lentils, chick peas, mung beans. If eating these are always best consumed sprouted	Fruit could be omitted earlier, but I feel that small amounts of fruit are seldom detrimental to health unless in the severely metabolically disordered	Sweet potato (kumara), yams, taro etc.
Use freely at any stage:						
Green Vegetables, pumpkin, peppers, herbs						
Eggs						
Butter, Ghee, coconut oil and extra virgin olive oil (all suitable for cooking)						
Macadamia, flax and hemp oils						
Meat, fish and poultry, tofu and tempeh						

Table 3. Carb-Appropriate food list. By the author.

**WHAT ABOUT DAIRY?

Dairy (especially milk) may be omitted if it is seen to trigger any GI, sinus, dermal or systemic symptoms. It is a common allergen, and there appears to be a rising incidence of milk protein intolerance and allergy.[151] I have often erred towards eliminating dairy early in the process of fat loss because of its highly insulinergic nature[152] and to help determine if the client does, in fact, have any degree of dairy protein intolerance or allergy.

The evidence though for the absolute avoidance of dairy by most people is sparse. In fact, in an adequate protein diet, a moderate dairy intake retains lean mass during dieting more effectively than the same protein with a lower dairy intake (and high protein, high dairy intake increases fat-loss).[153] People lose more fat when supplemented with calcium, and more again when the same amount of calcium is provided from a diary containing diet.[154, 155] It is likely to exert a synergistic effect along with dairy proteins (especially the BCAAs found in dairy in abundance) and angiotensin-converting enzyme inhibitors, to attenuate adiposity.[156]

Systematic reviews and meta-analyses of the evidence have concluded that increased dairy consumption without energy restriction or in long-term studies might not lead to a significant change in weight or body composition, but the inclusion of dairy in energy-restricted weight-loss diets significantly reduces weight, body-fat and improves lean-mass.[157, 158] There has also been demonstrated an inverse association between the intake of dairy products with type-2 diabetes[159, 160] and high-dairy consumption improves insulin resistance without negatively impacting bodyweight or cardiometabolic markers.[161]

Is there more to the dairy story?

The research typically looks at 'dairy' as a food group. Milk itself is (as previously mentioned) highly insulinergic and may, in contrast to the other dairy types (yoghurt, cheese, cottage cheese) still promote some adverse metabolic effects for some people. Milk can also be an interesting food-drink. Like alcohol, it can provide an additive or subtractive effect within the diet. This means that for some people a glass of milk will provide satiety and will reduce their consumption of food while others will simply drink milk in addition to their normal food intake and thus increase overall calorie intake. For these people eliminating milk could encourage further weight-loss.

Lactose in milk (or more specifically the galactose portion) is also a highly glycative sugar. In other words, it is one of the sugars (along with fructose) that has a high affinity to bind with proteins (such as proteins of artery walls, hormone receptor sites and others) causing them to become damaged and dysfunctional.

So should you remove diary?

My advice—use your best judgement. If you tolerate dairy proteins well, there is no good reason to avoid it. But if you feel that dairy promotes an intolerance or allergy reaction then avoid it for two weeks and see if you feel any better, then resume eating it for two weeks and notice any return of symptoms or lack thereof.

PROGRESSING THROUGH A STEP-WISE PROCESS

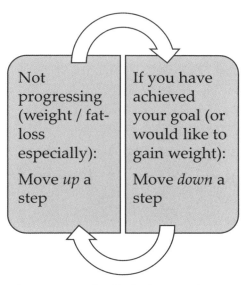

Not progressing (weight / fat-loss especially):	If you have achieved your goal (or would like to gain weight):
Move *up* a step	Move *down* a step

Figure 5. Progression strategy for Carb-Appropriate nutrition

As you move through a step-wise restriction, it is extremely easy to know whether to restrict further, continue to do what you're doing, or relax a little. If you are not losing weight, for example, you would want to take a further step UP (eat fewer carbs). If you have lost all the weight you'd like to lose, you could either stay where you are or step DOWN (to allow a little more carbohydrate). At any step though it is important to give yourself enough time to adjust and adapt to the changes you are putting in place. I suggest waiting at least two weeks at any stage in the process before moving up or down.

GOAL	Outcome of bi-weekly measurement		
	Weight Loss	**No Change**	**Weight Gain**
Weight Loss	Stay	↑Step Up	↑Step Up
Weight Maintenance	↓Step Down	Stay	↑Step Up
Weight Gain	↓Step Down	↓Step Down	Stay

Table 4. Carb-Appropriate step-wise progress matrix

Every two weeks or so progress can be re-evaluated. The matrix above you will further help you to know whether to stay, increase or decrease food categories according to the step-wise approach.

PLANT-BASED CARB-APPROPRIATE

Carb-Appropriate allows for significant variation and choice of food and so if you choose to abstain from meat (and other animal products) the method will still work perfectly well for you. Carb-Appropriate is a lower-carb diet in general (although not necessarily) and therefore, it could be wrongly equated with one that encourages a high meat intake.

It doesn't.

Many people prioritise the meat on their plates, to the detriment of vegetables and healthy oils. Think about the last time you went out for dinner and you, or someone else ordered a steak. Was it the 100, 120 or 150 g steak that would fulfil your protein requirements? Or was it the 300-400 g behemoth that for many would meet recommended protein amounts for the day *in a single meal?*

Complete abstinence from meat is not any healthier than an omnivorous diet, but it can be a great option for some. One thing I do like about a plant-based diet of any kind, whether it is vegan, vegetarian or simply a healthy omnivorous diet, is the focus on vegetables, which we could all stand to eat more. For this reason, I often recommend a plant-based diet for a short time in order to fall back in love with veggies!

In a balanced, healthy diet there is unlikely to be an excess of meat, especially if people are prioritising vegetables and trying to eat a minimum of three fist-sized servings per meal.

Carb-Appropriate for vegans and vegetarians requires just little more 'juggling'. Legumes for example (a great vegetarian protein source) should be eliminated as a last resort, or more likely not at all. Fruits and tubers could still be eliminated but in reality, an ad-libitum (eat as much as you want) vegan diet based on the Carb-Appropriate foundational principles of natural, whole and unprocessed food is likely to provide fantastic results anyway.

Those following a vegan diet should supplement with Vitamin B12. There is no reliable natural vegan source of B12 (except perhaps novel foods like Nori),[162, 163] and to prevent later neural damage from a B12 deficiency, it is always prudent to supplement.

WHAT ELSE IS GOING ON?

It is important to remember that many factors other than diet are important to performing well and living optimally. Other factors to consider are:

- Sleep quality
- Physical performance
- Cognition
- Mood
- Pain

If you feel any of these are worsening consult with a suitably qualified health practitioner.

CHAPTER 8

GOOD BUGS

Nutrition, health and the human microbiome

There is a lot of talk, and a lot of disinformation about 'gut health'. The 'gut' broadly refers to the entire gastro-oesophageal and gastrointestinal (GI) tract. The GI tract, although 'internal' in the sense that it is housed within the visceral cavity, is, in fact, an external organ. The various oesophageal, gastric, intestinal and anal sphincters are valves that close off the GI tract to the outside world, but it is in many respects similar to our skin, in that it is exposed to pathogens, environmental chemicals and of course specifically the food we eat. In that sense, it represents an 'external' tissue that is housed within the body.

The GI tract has a unique role in that it is equal parts a defender, repelling the things that we don't want and also a 'receiver' of the nutrients that we do want to sustain life. This unique combination of functions requires that the entire GI tract is working effectively to ensure that the right things enter the body (nutrients)...and other compounds such as potential toxins (toxicants) and pathogenic microbes are ejected.

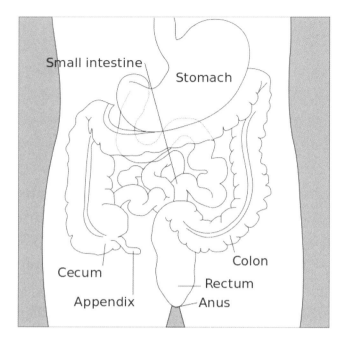

Figure 6. The human gastrointestinal tract.

THE MICROBIOME

The terms microbiome and microbiota are generally used synonymously, although technically the microbiome refers to the collective genomes of the organisms, whereas the microbiota refers to the organisms themselves. For simplicity, we will use the terms interchangeably.

The human body contains well over ten times more microbial cells than human cells accounting for up to 3% of our total body-mass. These 'non-human' cells include over 10,000 varieties of bacteria, viruses, protozoa, prions and bacteriophages with over eight million unique, protein-coding genes (in comparison to our 22,000).[164] These various organisms that we house have co-evolved with since the beginning of time and we have reached a level of symbiosis, which by definition means that we need them, and they us. Suffice it to say that having a healthy balance of gut flora is essential to optimal health, body-composition and performance.

The role of the microbiome in immunity and broader aspects of systemic health was largely ignored up until the 1990s. It is now suggested that the microbiome, and specifically having the 'right' balance of bacteria and the general health of the gut may play a much larger role that was previously believed in the expression of allergies, along with auto-immune diseases, obesity and metabolic disorders, brain diseases, psychological disorders and even cancer.

POPULATION OF THE GUT WITH BENEFICIAL BACTERIA

The majority of the initial population of the gut with beneficial bacteria occurs with the baby's passage down the vaginal canal during birth. This is our very first probiotic. Natural birth (vs. Caesarean birth) has been demonstrated to promote a better balance of intestinal flora and babies born by C-section have less bacterial diversity and a seeming absence of beneficial bifidobacteria.[165] They also have lower levels of lactobacillus and other intestinal bacteria and instead exhibit higher levels of bacteria typically associated with the microbiota of the skin (i.e. staphylococcus bacteria).[166] Babies born by C-section recover gut bacteria levels much more slowly than naturally born babies after administration of antibiotics to the mother during the birthing process,[167] creating a longer time to populate a 'normal' microbiota.[168]

Caesarean birth is associated with an increased risk of developing Coeliac Disease,[169] allergic rhinitis and possibly asthma,[170, 171] and a seven-fold increase in developing food allergies.[172]

There are clear health effects resulting from Caesarean birth, but in the perinatal period other factors such as the diet and lifestyle of the parents, environment, subsequent diet, use of antibiotics and whether the pregnancy was carried to full-term, play interrelated roles in health. It is not our place to judge Caesarean birth harshly as it is a medical necessity for many women. As we shall see the diet and lifestyle of the child can dictate the development of the microbiota and what role it goes on to play in long-term health.

PRO- AND PREBIOTICS: NATURAL COMPONENTS OF THE HUMAN DIET

Human breast milk is known to include lactobacillus species as well as other bacteria such as bifidobacteria. These are thought to originate in the gut and are transferred to the neonate via an enteromammary pathway. This pathway allows bacteria from the gut to be transported by way of immune cells (white blood cells) to the breast milk. This serves to further populate the digestive tract of the baby with good bacteria, boosting immunity and aiding the proper growth and development of the GI tract itself. Human milk also harbours a broad range of oligosaccharide prebiotics that promotes growth and activity of beneficial bacterial populations.[173, 174]

Attempts have been made to mimic this pre- and probiotic activity of breast milk. Prebiotic supplementation added to formula increases the number of bifidobacteria to a level comparable to breastmilk and reduces the pathogenic bacteria *Clostridium dificile*.[175] Inulin (a prebiotic fibre) has demonstrated efficacy in increasing bifidobacteria in the gut.[176] This is great news for women who have not been able to give birth naturally or who have chosen to formula-feed most, or all, of the time. A natural birth and breastfeeding are still considered to be the best option for both Mum and baby, but this is not always able to be done. A host of factors (that are beyond the scope of this book) determines the manner of feeding. The good news is that pre- and probiotic supplementation offer improved outcomes for babies and children that require formula-feeding.

PREBIOTICS IN TRADITIONAL DIETS

Prebiotics are resistant starches and fibres. They are so-called because they resist digestion in the gastrointestinal tract and are instead metabolised by gut bacteria, resulting in the proliferation of a health-promoting microbiota balance and the additional benefit of increased short-chain fatty acid (SFA) production. SFAs are utilised as fuel by other beneficial bacteria, leading to an 'upward cycle' of positive effects, and they can also be absorbed and used by the body as a priority fuel source. Interestingly it is these short chain fats that provide the majority of fuel for our closest relatives amongst the great apes. Gorillas, for example, derive the vast majority of their calories from these short chain fats which are produced in the gut, which in the case of these apes is a veritable power-house of voracious, fibre consuming bacteria!

Resistant starches and fibres are found in many vegetables, tubers, fruits, berries and grains. It is assumed that a diet based around natural, whole and unprocessed foods provides a range and quantity of these fibres that is conducive to optimised gut-health. Some processed foods (such as cornflakes) also provide resistant starch (RS) in the form of a 'retrograde' starch. This results from structural changes induced by cooking and cooling. However, one must be aware that these foods, while containing some RS also contain large amounts of fast-digesting carbohydrate that may overload your particular tolerance and thus promote weight-gain. For all but the most carb-tolerant individuals, my advice is to get your RS from natural, whole-foods!

Natural Resistant Starch			
Food	Serving size	Resistant starch (grams)	Carbohydrate content (grams)
Banana, raw, slightly green	1 medium, peeled	4.7	27
Oats, rolled	1/4 cup, uncooked	4.4	26
Green peas, frozen	1 cup, cooked	4.0	18
White beans	1/2 cup, cooked	3.7	23
Lentils	1/2 cup cooked	2.5	20
Cold potato	½ medium	0.6 - 0.8	19

Table 5. Natural sources of resistant starch.

Residual amounts of fibres and resistant starches are to be found in the lower-carbohydrate vegetables too. For those needing to follow lower-carb diets, the above options may provide too much glycaemic load and are thus unsuitable. In these cases, the naturally occurring fibres and starches from vegetables and berries are likely to be sufficient to aid gut health.

PROBIOTICS IN TRADITIONAL DIETS

Probiotics result from lactic acid fermentation of foods by bacteria. This process is a natural occurring one and foods containing these organisms have always been part of the diet of the modern man, *Homo sapiens*.[177] Lactic acid bacteria proliferate (albeit in small amounts) on foodstuffs that were eaten by our hunter-gatherer, and later, forebears.

Traditional diets likewise often contain foods with even higher concentrations of lactic acid bacteria. These foods have been developed as a way of preserving foods. This interesting symbiosis has served to not just preserve food for use, but to help preserve and maintain a healthy microbiome. Some of these traditional foods include kimchi, sauerkraut, pickles, naturally prepared olives and other preserved vegetables and fruits, cultured butter, yoghurt and kefir. All of these foods provide a valuable addition to the diet and we should strive to incorporate at least one serve of cultured food per day to our diet.

POOR GUT HEALTH – WHAT IS A 'LEAKY GUT'?

Alessio Fasano—one of the leading researchers in the field of the human microbiome, has suggested that one of the under-recognised factors in the expression of autoimmune diseases is increased intestinal permeability.[178] The role of a 'leaky gut' in other more insidious conditions (such as fatigue, depression and general feelings of malaise and poor wellbeing) are not well understood, but there is evidence that a leaky gut affects a host of systems and negatively affects many health conditions. For example, it has been suggested that leaky gut plays a role in the development of cancer.[179] In autoimmune intestinal diseases, increased intestinal permeability encourages diarrhoea via a 'leak-flux' mechanism, and in conjunction with this, other junctions are altered and lumen uptake of macromolecules is enhanced.[180] Interestingly *faecal calprotectin* (a marker of disease activity in the inflammatory bowel diseases such as Crohn's Disease) also indicates leaky gut in Alzheimer's Disease.[181]

Impaired intestinal integrity may also promote diabetes via an autoimmune mechanism affecting the beta cells of the pancreas and through increased inflammation that encourages insulin resistance.[182]

A leaky-gut is directly correlated with liver disorders and the inflammatory process resulting from a leaky gut are thought to contribute to alcoholic and non-alcoholic liver diseases.[183-186]

Many bacteria within the gut contain lipopolysaccharides (LPS) within their outer membranes. LPS elicits a strong immune response, endotoxaemia (internal toxicity symptoms) and systemic inflammation which may be associated with cardiovascular disease,[187] autoimmune conditions,[188, 189] and depression.[190] As bacteria are destroyed by an immune response, or simply die off naturally, LPS can be taken up into the body via a leaky-gut. Animal research (in mice) suggests that LPS is a causative factor for obesity, insulin resistance and diabetes[191-193] and correlation is now beginning to be demonstrated in human subjects between LPS induced endotoxaemia and obesity.[194]

PROBIOTIC THERAPY

Probiotics are extremely popular supplements, but much of the research is still in its infancy. They certainly hold a lot of promise and are a valuable addition to the diet to help support the balance of bacteria in the gut.

- Supplements of *Lactobacillus rhamnosus* types positively change gut bacteria.[195]
- Taking these supplements in early infancy also has long-term postive effects on the microbiota composition.[195, 196]
- It has also been suggested that probiotic supplements support nutrient status (especially folate and B12 levels) in those with greater levels of inflammation.[197]
- Probiotics (in this case in the form of a probiotic 'biscuit') have been shown effective in redressing some of the age-related dysbiosis of the intestinal microbiota. In particular, the probiotic treatment reverted the age-related increase of the opportunistic pathogens *Clostridium* cluster XI, *Clostridium difficile*, *C. perfringens*, *Enterococcus faecium* and the enteropathogenic genus *Campylobacter* that cause diarrhoea and malabsorption in the elderly.[198]

- *E. coli* Nissle 1917 increases expression of proteins responsible for improving gut integrity (ZO-1)and reduces intestinal permeability in mice with experimentally induced colitis.[199]

There is more, and emerging research suggests a compelling positive role for probiotic supplements as an addition to the diet, especially in those who were born by Caesarean section, have had extensive antibiotic treatment or don't regularly eat fermented foods.

NUTRIENTS AND GUT HEALTH

B VITAMINS

B Vitamins help to improve the integrity of the intestinal wall. One of the protective actions of niacin (vitamin B3) may be that it increases junction proteins in the gut.[200]

GLUTAMINE

A gut healing protocol including glutamine, NAC and zinc attenuates IgA and IgM immune responses to LPS in those with chronic fatigue syndrome.[201]

ZINC

Zinc supplementation (110 mg zinc sulphate, three times per day) may improve intestinal permeability in those with Crohn's Disease.[202]

TIPS FOR IMPROVING GUT HEALTH

- Eat a natural, unprocessed diet
  A naturally based diet is likely to be higher in fibres and resistant starches beneficial for gut-health along with micro-nutrients beneficial for preserving the integrity of the gut wall and of gut function generally.

- Take a supportive multi-nutrient formula daily
  As many of us are lacking one or more of the essential vitamins or minerals from diet alone supplementing with a quality multi-nutrient formula helps to ensure 'nutritional insurance' for gut (and systemic) health.

- Eat traditional, fermented foods at every meal
  Without creating a lot of stress and worry about what to take and how much, simply try to introduce fermented foods, according to taste and tolerability at any meals that you can. These will help to subtly 'seed' the gut with beneficial bacteria, and regular use will aid the maintenance of these beneficial populations.

- Use purified (unchlorinated water)
  Chlorinated water *may* reduce beneficial bacteria. This may not eventually be proven effective, but the beneficial effect of the chlorine (reduction of harmful bacteria) has already been realised by the time water reaches your glass, and so there is no god reason to NOT use water with the chlorine removed.

- Take probiotics as needed

Probiotic supplements can be used routinely and regularly or irregularly depending on the degree of support your gut requires. A suitably qualified practitioner can help to determine the best type, dosage and frequency for you.

PROBIOTIC SUPPLEMENTATION: GENERAL RECOMMENDATIONS

Specific recommendations for disease or disorder should always be made by a practitioner, however for those of us wishing to reap some of the potential benefits of improved gut health a broader supportive strategy (compared to a focused, therapeutic strategy) can be the best option. Look for a supplement that includes at least 30 billion CFU of a range of probiotics including the following:

- *Lactobacillus plantarum* (found in kimchi)
- *L. brevis* (found in sauerkraut and pickles)
- *L. acidophilus, Bifidobacterium lactis/animalis* (found in yoghurt and kefir)
- And *L. rhamnosus, B. longum, L. reuteri*

THE EMERGING SCIENCE OF FAECAL TRANSPLANTS

Faecal transplants are beginning to be investigated as a way of correcting the microbiome. This procedure is either fascinating or disgusting depending on your point of view and usually involves the transplanting of faecal matter from a healthy donor, into the bowel of someone with a health condition.

- Reviews of 11 studies with 273 participants suggest that faecal microbiota transplants are effective for resolving *Clostridium dificile* infection (CDI),[203] a common cause of diarrhoea and colitis. However, there is a paucity of randomised controlled trials to fully confirm this initial finding.
- A 2015 review including 45 studies suggests a curative effect is likely for CDI, Ulcerative Colitis (UC), and Irritable Bowel Syndrome (IBS) but not for Crohn's Disease (CD) or pouchitis.
- One RCT demonstrated a significant improvement in metabolic syndrome.[204]
- Another review of 18 studies (nine cohort studies, eight case studies and one randomized controlled trial) of 122 patients with ulcerative colitis (UC) or Crohn's disease (CD) found that 45% of patients achieved remission during follow-up. Among the cohort studies, clinical remission was achieved in 36.2% people.[205]

More research is required to better understand the application and benefits of faecal transplants, but they offer an interesting and plausible treatment option for a range of disorders.

CHAPTER 9

SUPPLEMENTATION

A step-wise approach to supplementation for maximum benefit at minimum cost

Supplementation, like the rest of your nutrition, should be approached in a 'do only what you must' manner. All too often when people seek advice from a complementary health provider they are prescribed a plethora of supplements at great cost and with the considerable hassle of having to remember when to take them all. On the one hand, there's nothing wrong with prescribing supplements to the diet (I do it regularly) if they are going to benefit the client, but finding the most effective supplement strategy, at the lowest cost and with the minimum of fuss should be the paramount concern.

Supplementation needs to be both efficacious and easy, because if it's not it will not be sustainable. Much research around supplementation is certainly lacking and many supplements offer more hype than hope. As mentioned earlier, many of us do not get all that we need from diet alone, in particular, the vitamins A, B1, B6, B12, iron (especially women), zinc (especially important for men), and selenium—which nearly half of all New Zealanders do not consume in adequate amounts. The data showing that we lack nutrients from our diets are based on minimum daily requirements (not on what is optimal). Optimal amounts of some vitamins and minerals are significantly higher than the Nutrient Reference Values (NRV) Dietary Recommended Intakes (DRI). With so many diets lacking essential nutrients, and in order to perform at our best it makes sense to support the body with intelligent supplementation.

VITAMINS AND MINERALS IN BRIEF

VITAMIN B1

Thiamin (B1) (or *thiamine*) was the first B vitamin discovered (hence it is B '1'). It is required by every cell to produce energy (ATP). The heart requires a particularly high amount of thiamin and many symptoms of deficiency are related to impaired heart function. Along with its generally supportive role for the heart and general health, at least one randomised controlled trial suggests that vitamin B1 improves mental function.[206]

VITAMIN B2

Riboflavin (B2) is critical to the body's production of its main energy source adenosine triphosphate (ATP). It aids the processing of amino acids and fat and activates vitamin B6 and folate.

Riboflavin is thought to help reduce migraines.[207]

VITAMIN B3

Vitamin B3 is required for the proper functioning of more than 50 enzymes and many chemical reactions throughout the body. It helps to release energy from both fats and carbohydrates and is involved in hormone production. It may help to support cardiovascular health and blood sugar regulation.

VITAMIN B5

Vitamin B5 aids the making of proteins (the building blocks of cells, organs and tissue) and helps to metabolise fats and carbohydrates. It also supports the production of various hormones and red blood cells.

VITAMIN B6

Vitamin B6 aids the production of proteins, hormones and neurotransmitters. Mild B6 deficiencies are common in children and it is recommended to supplement this vitamin.[208]

VITAMIN B9 (FOLATE)

Folate, also known as Vitamin B9, plays a critical role in many biological processes. It is involved in the crucial process of methylation and also plays a vital role in cell division (the fundamental process of growth and development). Adequate folate is needed to support heart health, prevent birth defects and support proper growth and development.

It is important to use an active methylated form of folate; L5 methyltetrahydrafolate (L5MTHF) in preference to the cheaper synthetic form often simply labelled 'folic acid'. Many people cannot effectively convert other synthetic forms of folic acid to active folate in the body. The common synthetic form of folic acid (pteroylmonoglutamate) found in most supplements leads to high levels of unmetabolised folic acid in the blood.[209, 210] This can interfere with the function of active folate,[211, 212] negatively affecting immunity.[213] (Discussed in Appendix B)

VITAMIN C

Humans, unlike most mammals, (but interestingly in common with bats and guinea pigs) can't make Vitamin C and so we need to eat foods containing this vitamin regularly. Vitamin C is a key antioxidant and is crucial for the formation of collagen (connective tissue).

A Cochrane database review of the evidence suggests that regular Vitamin C supplementation can reduce the length and severity of the common cold.[214]

VITAMIN D

Vitamin D is a vitamin that acts like a hormone. It is involved with bone deposition, immune and inflammatory regulation and mood. Cholecalciferol Vitamin D3 has been demonstrated in a Cochrane review to improve mortality.

Good news for our vegetarian and vegan friends is that there is now Vitamin D3 derived from lichen (previously the most widely available D3 was extracted from sheep's wool).

VITAMIN E

Vitamin E is a family of fat-soluble, antioxidant vitamins. While research is mixed, it suggests that having a diet high in Vitamin E and other antioxidants is supportive for cardiovascular and general health.

Emerging research suggests the best results may come from using mixed tocopherols and tocotrienols to provide the broadest range of health supporting effects. It has been suggested that only using the common (alpha-tocopherol) form reduces levels of other health promoting forms of Vitamin E (such as gamma-tocopherol).[215]

VITAMIN K

Vitamin K plays an important role in promoting proper coagulation and wound healing. It is also involved in regulating immunity and inflammation and in aiding proper bone construction and development.

BIOTIN

Biotin (sometimes known as Vitamin B7) is a water soluble vitamin that plays an important role in metabolizing the energy we derive from carbohydrates, proteins and fats.

Vitamin B12

Vitamin B12 (cobalamin) is required for proper functioning of nerve cells and works in conjunction with Vitamin B6 and folate to reduce levels of homocysteine (high levels of homocysteine are linked to a wide range of health problems). Without adequate B12 people can suffer from a form of anaemia and ultimately a lack of B12 can damage neurons. As B12 is predominantly found in animal foods, vegetarians and especially vegans are at a greater risk of deficiency and it is recommended that these populations take a daily B12 supplement as a preventative measure to reduce the risk of severe neural damage later in life.

Look for the methylcobalamin and adenosylcobalamin forms of B12 in supplements as these are the bioactive forms naturally occurring in the human body.

Copper

Copper is an essential trace mineral that is a vital component of many enzymes.

Chromium

Chromium helps the body to regulate blood sugar. Chromium is a co-factor for the actions of insulin—the hormone that aids the transport of blood sugar into cells.

IRON

As a component of haemoglobin (the oxygen carrying protein found in red blood cells) and myoglobin (which stores oxygen in muscle), iron is crucial to preserve oxygen delivery and availability, and thereby crucial for energy creation. Iron deficiency can lead to anaemia, learning disabilities, impaired immune function, fatigue, and depression. Iron overload is relatively common and so you shouldn't supplement with iron unless advised by a physician after appropriate testing is carried out.

MANGANESE

Manganese is a mineral only required in trace amounts but is important as a component of many enzymes. Manganese plays an important role as part of the antioxidant enzyme superoxide dismutase (SOD), which helps combat free radicals. It is also involved in supporting energy metabolism, thyroid function, blood glucose control and skeletal growth.

MAGNESIUM

Magnesium is an essential mineral. It is used for many functions throughout the body including muscle relaxation, blood clotting and the manufacture of ATP (the cells fuel). It is considered to be generally relaxing due to its relationship with calcium. It reduces hyper-excitability of neurons.

Magnesium supplements can reduce the incidence of migraines,[216, 217] menstrual migraines,[218] and headaches.[219] Magnesium supplements may help prevent noise related hearing damage.[220]

Magnesium works in conjunction with potassium and calcium to reduce over-active nerve firing and this influences arterial blood pressure. Magnesium supplementation can reduce high blood pressure,[221,222, 223] reduce menstrual pain,[224] help dysmenorrhoea in general[225] and reduce symptoms of PMS.[226, 227]

SILICA

Silicon helps the body to produce collagen (connective tissue) and supports the health of skin, hair and nails.

However, the *orthosilicic acid* form of silicon is the only form that has demonstrated benefits for the health of skin, hair and nails in research trials.[228]

POTASSIUM

Potassium is an essential mineral and one of our major electrolytes. Potassium works hand in hand with sodium to preserve proper transmission of nerve signals and for proper fluid balance. Potassium supplementation helps those with high blood pressure. A meta-analysis of randomised controlled trials found that potassium supplements reduce blood pressure, especially in those eating too much salt.[229]

SELENIUM

Selenium is a trace mineral that the body uses to produce glutathione peroxidase, an integral part of the body's antioxidant defence system. It works with Vitamin E to protect cell membranes. It's also essential for proper thyroid hormone regulation and metabolism as Selenium is a co-factor in the conversion of the thyroid hormone thyroxine (T4) to the more active form triiodothyronine (T3).

ZINC

Zinc is a mineral involved in many chemical reactions throughout the body. It is considered to be extremely immune supporting. A Cochrane Database review of randomised controlled trials suggests specific benefits that include; reducing the symptoms of the common cold and respiratory infections,[230] and reduced rates of persistent diarrhoea in children.[231] There is also preliminary evidence suggesting zinc supplementation may help to reduce symptoms of ADHD in children.[232]

ANTIOXIDANTS

Free radicals are highly unstable molecules that can damage cell membranes and DNA (genetic information) in cells. The normal functions of the human body produce some free radicals, and free radical formation is accelerated in response to high sun exposure, tobacco smoke, sunlight, X-rays, and a poor diet. Antioxidants are substances that inactivate 'free radicals'. To combat free radicals, the body utilises antioxidants to reduce the potential for excessive cell damage.

Current Nutrient Reference Values for Recommended Dietary Intakes in New Zealand and Australia can be found at https://www.nrv.gov.au/nutrients

NATURAL OR SYNTHETIC SUPPLEMENTS?

Many people make the assumption that 'natural' supplements must be superior, or must be more easily absorbed, digested or metabolised. This is not necessarily true, and in this case, it is fair to say that the devil is in the details.

If a vitamin or mineral is an identical form whether it is synthesised in the lab or extracted from food, then on a molecular level it is exactly the same. So for example, ascorbic acid (Vitamin C) is ascorbic acid whether from a plant or from the lab. It is much cheaper and more efficient to create large amounts of Vitamin C in the lab and so when you see Vitamin C in a product you can almost always assume that it has been created…AND that it is every bit as good as Vitamin C found in foods. However, what it does not contain are the natural cofactors (like bioflavonoids) that help it to more appropriately do its job of reducing oxidative damage in the body. Often the advantage of using vitamins and minerals from natural, whole-food sources is not because of any particular vitamin or mineral itself, but instead because of the *range* of co-operating nutrients contained within.

Sometimes though (and this is why the devil is in the details!) what is called Vitamin X is not the same as something else called Vitamin X.

This is particularly of relevance to for example folic acid vs. 'folate'. While technically interchangeable these terms in common usage refer to quite different chemicals that have very different effects on the body, likewise for the more common cyanocobalamin form of B12, which is less effective than the naturally occurring methyl- and adenosylcobalamin forms. Some forms of vitamins especially may be less effective or even potentially harmful (for a subset of the population).

	Common or Less Effective Form	Preferable Form
Vitamin B9	Pteroylmonoglutamate ('folic acid')	L-5 methyltetrahydrafolate
Vitamin B12	Cyanocobalamin	Methyl- and/or adenosylcobalamin
Vitamin C	Ascorbic acid	Ascorbic acid with natural bioflavonoids
Vitamin D	Ergocalciferol (D2)	Cholecalciferol (D3)
Vitamin E	Isolated alpha-tocopherol	Mixed tocopherols and tocotrienols
Vitamin K	Phylloquinone (K1)	Mixed K1 and K2 (menaquinone) especially menaquinone-7 (K2-MK7)

Table 6. Preferred forms of supplemental vitamins.

BEWARE 'GREEN ALLOPATHY'

The term 'green allopathy' is one that describes the system employed by many naturopaths and nutritionists in which they treat symptoms with a plethora of supplements, herbs or other modality remedies. Notwithstanding that I don't believe this is even what naturopathy or clinical nutrition should be, it can also lead to over-prescription and this can (even if sub-consciously) be driven by a commercial imperative. It absolutely grinds my gears when I see someone walking out of a naturopath's office with hundreds (and sometimes thousands) of dollars' worth of pills and potions when simple dietary and lifestyle interventions could have provided a more credible, cost-effective solution. In many cases, one or two supplements in addition to a good lifestyle and nutrition plan will be as effective as or more so than a range of specific application supplements cobbled together. Let's face it, *nutrition* involves foods that are bundles of many thousands of micro- and macronutrients. The body is very well developed to absorb, metabolise and utilise these nutrients and it is naïve to think that the same cannot be done from real, whole-food based supplements.

There obviously is a place for specific-application supplementation, but not before or in the place of better whole-food interventions, and broad-based supplementation that supports general nutrient requirements.

A STEP-WISE GUIDE TO SUPPLEMENTATION

There is a place for supplementation for general health (i.e. apart from treating frank or sub-clinical deficiencies) and a step-wise approach similar to what we employed for diet can also be used to determine what is going to give you the best 'bang-for-your-buck' when deciding which supplements to take.

STEPWISE SUPPLEMENTATION

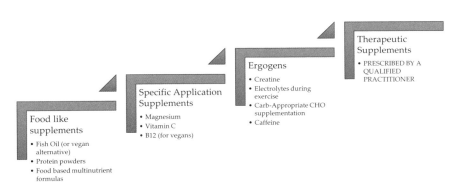

Figure 7. A step-wise approach to supplementation.

STEP 1: FOOD-LIKE SUPPLEMENTS

At the base of our step-wise approach to supplementation are foods or food extracts that help to provide nutrients that we may otherwise lack in our diets. Primary among these is omega-3 supplementation, food-based multi-nutrients and protein powders.

FISH OIL

Omega-3 (n-3) fats and Omega-6 (n-6) fats contain the essential fats and their metabolites that are the key modulators of inflammatory function. Excessive inflammation has been suggested as a causative factor in a host of illnesses including autoimmune conditions, diabetes and insulin resistance, heart disease, cancer and neurological (brain) disorders. It is suggested that the balance of n-3 to n-6 fats should be one part to less than seven parts. Our modern, western-style diet has a disproportionate amount of n-6 fats that is pro-inflammatory. By emphasising whole foods and reducing intake of refined seed oils, processed foods (that include high n-6 fats) in general, and factory farmed meats and eggs (which are also higher in n-6 fats and lower in n-3 fats), we can redress this imbalance.

Supplementation of n-3 fat containing oils is likely to offer additional benefits and this is especially true of fish oil.

Fish oil supplementation is likely to be generally cardioprotective[233] and has several positive effects on health markers such as reducing triglycerides in a dose-dependent manner,[234, 235] increasing HDL cholesterol and the HDL to LDL ratio,[236] and reducing blood pressure.[237] The effect on blood pressure (reduction of approximately 2.5 mm/Hg and 1.5 mm/Hg for systolic and diastolic blood pressure respectively) is similar to that observed when salt intake is drastically reduced. Evidence also suggests that increased consumption of n–3 FAs from fish or fish-oil supplements reduces rates of all-cause mortality, cardiac and sudden death, and possibly stroke.[238, 239] A 2012 systematic review published in the *Journal of the American Medical Association* concluded that there was little significant effect from n-3 PUFA supplementation, however generally favourable results were observed across studies for all cause and cardiovascular mortality.[240]

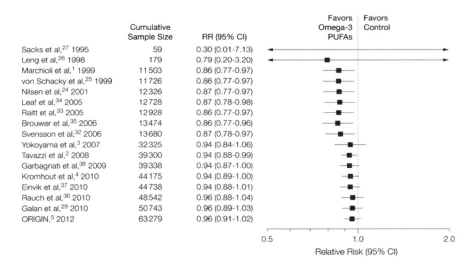

Figure 8. Association Between Omega-3 Fatty Acid Supplementation and Risk of Major Cardiovascular Disease Events: A Systematic Review and Meta-analysis JAMA. 2012;308(10):1024-1033. doi:10.1001/2012.jama.11374

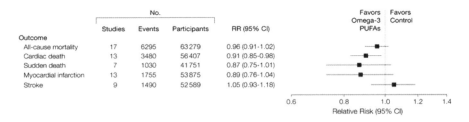

Figure 9. Association Between Omega-3 Fatty Acid Supplementation and Risk of Major Cardiovascular Disease Events: A Systematic Review and Meta-analysis JAMA. 2012;308(10):1024-1033. doi:10.1001/2012.jama.11374

These cardiometabolic benefits are not observed to the same degree from increased consumption of alpha-linolenic acid,[241] the 'base' omega-3 fat found in plant-derived sources such as flaxseed oil.

Benefits from fish oil supplementation are also seen in depression.[242, 243] A modest but consistent benefit from marine n-3 PUFAs is seen for joint swelling and pain, duration of morning stiffness, global assessments of pain and disease activity, and use of non-steroidal anti-inflammatory drugs in rheumatoid artritis.[244] Interestingly despite a compelling rationale (i.e. reduction in inflammation) we are yet to see insufficient evidence to suggest a protective role of n-3 supplementation in cancer and inflammatory bowel diseases, notwithstanding that there are compelling reasons to take (n-3) supplements for general health if we have these conditions.

Daily dose: 1.2-1.8 g DHA/EPA minimum (or approximately 4000 mg of fish oil)

WHAT ABOUT KRILL OIL?

DHA and EPA from Krill oil are taken up into plasma more effectively than those EFA metabolites from fish oil (around 80% vs. 60% respectively)[245] but large standard deviations in these results may make this not applicable on an individual level.

Similar positive effects on human blood lipid profiles and total body oxidation rates have been observed from Krill oil supplementation of 543 mg vs. 863 mg of EPA-DHA in Krill or Fish Oil respectively (in other words a Krill supplement with 62.8% the EPA-DHA amount of Fish Oil). This demonstrates a greater proportional effect from taking Krill Oil.[246]

What does this mean?

Krill oil is often promoted as a far superior alternative to fish oil but the evidence doesn't back up this claim. It's fair to say that because of higher uptake of DHA and EPA, that Krill Oil is more effective than Fish Oil of the same dose. Because of this around 3000 mg Krill Oil can be used instead of 4000 mg Fish Oil.

MULTINUTRIENT PRODUCTS

The common lack of nutrients in the modern diet (as evidenced by the micronutrient information referenced earlier) make it prudent to supplement with a multi-nutrient.

A multi-nutrient is never a substitute for good eating and *food always comes first* but a multi- can help to provide some of the things that we may habitually, or occasionally lack for optimal health and performance.

WHAT TO LOOK FOR IN A MULTINUTRIENT?

- Contains all the essential micronutrients—with the possible exception of iron because up to 20% or more of people may experience sub-clinical iron overload
- Based on whole-food ingredients and extracts that provide additional 'secondary' nutrients
- Uses the safest and most effective forms of ingredients
- Doesn't contain ingredients simply because they are 'trending' or popular if they don't have evidence to support safety and efficacy

WHOLE FOOD INGREDIENTS

Whole-foods including herbs, berries, vegetables (and their respective extracts) help to provide 'secondary nutrients'. These nutrients are antioxidant (and other) compounds that help to support health in addition to the essential micro-nutrients. Conventionally farmed produce is often lacking in secondary nutrients produce and they are not typically found in appreciable amounts in highly processed and refined food items. (See Appendix C for a list of some of these whole-food ingredients)

SAFEST AND MOST EFFECTIVE FORMS TO LOOK FOR:

PREFORMED VITAMIN A PLUS MIXED CAROTENOIDS FOR ENHANCED EFFECTS

The most commonly used carotenoid in supplements is beta-carotene, a vegetable derived carotenoid that is converted into active Vitamin A. However conversion rates of beta-carotene to usable Vitamin A differ by a factor of nine-fold[247] and beta-carotene is required in amounts at least four times higher than pre-formed Vitamin A.[248, 249] For this reason, both preformed Vitamin A (for example from retinyl palmitate) along with sufficient beta-carotene (pro-vitamin A) and other naturally occurring carotenoids help to ensure optimal Vitamin A levels to get the full range of its health effects.

BETTER FORMS OF B12

The common form added to supplements, *cyanocobalamin,* is a synthetic form not found naturally in foods. The metabolism of cyanocobalamin leaves behind a cyanide residue that the body must then excrete. This is unlikely to cause problems for most people (the amount of cyanide left is extremely small) but it has been suggested that those with pre-existing kidney problems may have trouble excreting even these small amounts and that a methylcobalamin form is preferred.[250] For decades now it has been recommended that cyanocobalamin should be replaced with a non-cyanide form of B12 for general safety.[251] Naturally occurring cobalamins (like methylcobalamin) in food are also absorbed more effectively than synthetic B12 (cyanocobalamin).[252, 253]

An alternative to synthetic vitamin B12 is a natural co-factor of B12, *methylcobalamin.* Vitamin B12 regulates, together with 5-methyl-tetrahydrofolic acid (folate), the remethylation of homocysteine to l-methionine and the subsequent formation of S-adenosylmethionine (SAMe). SAMe is essential to most biological methylation reactions including the methylation of myelin, neurotransmitters, and phospholipids (e.g. phosphatidylcholine).

Methylcobalamin, having a methyl group is able to act as a methyl donor for these reactions,[254] whereas the synthetic forms need to themselves be methylated in order to do this. This step may be limited in some people and even in healthy people could tax methylation pathways unnecessarily.

GREAT LEVELS OF B VITAMINS

B vitamins are essential for the creation of fuel within cells and a host of enzyme reactions within the body. Kids Good Stuff provides more B vitamins than the leading multi-nutrient formulas for kids.

A BETTER FORM OF B9

Always choose supplements with the active methylated forms of folate such as L5-methyltetrahydrafolate (L5MTHF) in preference to the cheaper synthetic form often simply labelled 'folic acid'. Many people cannot effectively convert synthetic forms (like pteroylmonoglutamate) of folic acid to active folate in the body. This can lead to high levels of unmetabolised folic acid in the blood,[209, 210] that in turn interferes with the functions of active folate,[211, 212] negatively affecting immunity[213] and creating a possible tumourgenic (cancer causing) stimulus. (See Appendix B for more information on folate versus folic acid)

BROAD SPECTRUM VITAMIN E SUPPORT

It was once thought that the only active form of Vitamin E in the body was d-alpha-tocopherol. However, all four tocopherols and four tocotrienols are beginning to demonstrate important health functions, including increased antioxidant activity and reductions in cancer formation. Overloading with alpha-tocopherol alone may reduce levels of the other health-promoting forms of Vitamin E in the body.[215] Choose a mixed tocopherol/tocotrienol blend that also has ample amounts of alpha-tocopherol.

INCLUDES ESSENTIAL VITAMIN K

Commonly omitted from nutrient formulas, Vitamin K plays an important role in promoting proper coagulation and wound healing. It is also involved in regulating immunity and inflammation and in aiding proper bone construction and development.

Note: Vitamin K2, menaquinone-7 (K2-MK7) has demonstrated promise to help reduce arterial calcification and so may offer additional cardiovascular benefits.

INCLUDES ALPHA-LIPOIC ACID FOR INCREASED ANTIOXIDANT ACTION

Alpha lipoic acid is a type of fatty acid that's found in every cell and helps to generate energy. Alpha lipoic acid also functions as an antioxidant and unlike most antioxidants works in both water and fatty tissues and so has a broad spectrum of antioxidant actions.

SELENIUM TO SUPPORT THYROID HEALTH

Selenium is an important antioxidant mineral. It works with Vitamin E to protect cell membranes and is involved with proper thyroid function—by aiding the conversion of the thyroid hormone thyroxine (T4) to the more active form triiodothyronine (T3). It is extremely low in New Zealand soils and thus nearly half of New Zealanders do not get enough from diet alone.

STEP 2: SUPPORTIVE SPECIFIC APPLICATION SUPPLEMENTS

Some supplements are useful to support the modern lifestyle. It is a murky area because supplements, especially those that contain herbs, can be dangerous for people with certain conditions and when used with some medications. However, some supplements are effective and generally considered safe for people without health condition or taking medication.

MAGNESIUM

Commonly used to encourage better sleep and for relaxation purposes. Many people may be marginally deficient in this mineral and it is important for cardiovascular health.

ZINC

25% or more of the population are zinc deficient. It is one of the few supplements that may actually reduce the duration and severity of the common cold. Be aware though that zinc can become toxic if taken in high doses for too long. If in doubt always check with your health practitioner.

VITAMIN B12

Vegans and vegetarians can be at risk of B12 deficiency as there are no reliable sources of B12 in non-animal products. B12 deficiency can cause low energy, fatigue and in the long-term can cause significant neural damage. For this reason alone, it is always prudent for any vegan or vegetarian to supplement with B12 or a B12 containing multi- product.

VITAMIN C

Regular and consistent use of Vitamin C supplements can actually reduce the duration and severity of the common cold, however simply 'loading up' on Vitamin C when you get a cold is unlikely to do anything. Athletes and others under significant stress-load also benefit from the immune-boosting effects of Vitamin C.

Step 3: Ergogenic Supplements (Performance Enhancers)

Creatine

Creatine is considered the most effective ergogenic nutritional supplement currently available. Papers numbering in the thousands have now been published, with most showing positive benefits.

Creatine has been demonstrated to:

- Improve high-intensity exercise capacity
- Improve maximal strength and power
- Be safe when used by healthy populations

Recommendation:
0.3 g per kg bodyweight per day for five days followed by 5 g per day or 2-5 g per day

Electrolyte Drinks During Exercise

The only electrolyte proven to improve performance when taken during exercise is humble old sodium. We have already discussed how this essential mineral has been much derided by the standard dietary guidelines, but during exercise, its role is even more important. Sodium is a key regulator of fluid balance in the body. While the kidneys do a great job of regulating sodium levels at rest, so that if you take in too much your body will excrete more, and if you take in too little the body will excrete less, during exercise, this does not occur. We typically we don't pee during exercise and there is a significant difference observed in sodium excretion from the skin between individuals and this variation appears to be genetically mediated. So, if you happen to be one of those people who lose much more sodium in sweat, you may need to supplement with a sodium-containing electrolyte solution during exercise.

Make sure that the drink you choose is appropriate to your carb requirements though, as many are little more than sugar-water, and usually with insufficient sodium. An appropriate electrolyte drink would contain between 500 and 1000 mg of sodium per litre with little, if any, sugar. Carbs can always be added according to your own requirements.

Electrolyte	Typical daily intake (mg)	Typical absorption efficiency	Typical sweat losses per litre	Loss in litres of sweat to be deficient	Deficiency possible by sweating?
Sodium	4000	>90%	230-1700	4	Yes
Potassium	2700	>90%	150	16	No
Calcium	500	30%	28	5	Possible
Magnesium	300	10-70%	8.3-14.2	15	No

Table 7. Electrolyte intake, absorption and losses in sweat.

STEP 4: THERAPEUTIC SUPPLEMENTS AND HERBS

At this highest level, supplements can fall under the heading of *orthomolecular medicine*. This is the application of much larger (than normal) doses of a supplement (especially a vitamin or mineral) to offer a specific benefit to health conditions, or the application of a herb in sufficient dose to have a treatment effect. Because of the risks of drug-herb-food-supplement reactions, this should only ever be done by a qualified practitioner.

IMPORTANT NOTES ABOUT SUPPLEMENTATION

Clinical diagnosis of nutrient deficiencies is beyond the scope of this book. If you suspect a deficiency, you should check with a suitably qualified practitioner who can observe clinical signs and symptoms, and send you for further testing as required, and prescribe appropriate supplements for you.

If you have a health condition or are using prescribed medications seek appropriate health advice before using nutritional supplements and herbal medicines.

CHAPTER 10

QUANTIFYING

Getting specific with Carbohydrate-Appropriate nutrition

Quality always provides the base for a healthy diet. If we focus on natural, whole and unprocessed foods, we are more likely to ingest ample micronutrients and beneficial fibres and starches and are less likely to overload with either excessive carbohydrate or altered, harmful fat types (such as the majority of trans-fats[i]). In fact, as we have already discussed, most of us, most of the time can eat a natural, whole, unprocessed diet, *ad libitum* (eat as much as you like!) and not over-eat.

However, there are times when quantification is necessary. Athletes and those with health conditions can benefit from increased quantification and you may require a more quantified approach to nutrition if:

---

[i] Some fats that are technically trans-fats are considered healthy, including vaccenic acid from meat and dairy and many of the conjugated linoleic acid family

- You suffer from a metabolic disorder
- You are dieting heavily
- You are trying to put on large amounts of muscle
- Your sport performance is not currently optimised

QUANTIFYING CALORIES

It can be useful from time-to-time to evaluate how much you're eating. I really don't have a lot of love for calorie counting…but it can be a good exercise in understanding better how much food is required to fuel the body, and how different foods (and portion sizes) supply this fuel.

There are many ways to calculate calories. Most popular nowadays are the various apps and software available to both work out calories in the food you eat, and determining (but remembering that everybody is different) how many calories you need to consume for your goal. Be wary though as many of the default settings in these apps are geared towards 'best-practice' guidelines which are typically too high in carbohydrate and not high enough in either quality protein or healthy fats for the best achievement of many people's goals.

A good option for an app is *My Fitness Pal,* which is available for both Android and iPhone.

HPN certification members can also access clinical calorie calculators in the HPN Leaning Management System (see Appendix D for manual calculations of calories).

The average calorie requirement for males is 2200 without activity factors added in, and for women, this figure is 1800 calories.

QUANTIFYING MACRONUTRIENTS

How your calories are split up into the macros is determined by your goals, activity level, activity type and your unique metabolic tolerance.

Your own tolerance for carbohydrate will be influenced by your ethnicity, gender, age and what you have conditioned your body to prefer over many years and this will, in turn, affect how much relative fat and protein you should consume. For example, if you tolerated carbohydrate very well when you were younger, and consequently ate a lot of highly processed, highly refined, high carb-load foods you may begin to become less efficient over time and exhibit some of the symptoms of metabolic disorders. If this is the case, you would now be predisposed to a diet that is lower in carbohydrate. However, (and I can't state this enough) there is no one-size-fits-all, and some people WILL do well over their entire lifetime on a higher-carb diet!

There are several ways to split up the amounts of macronutrients in the diet.

		Protein	Carbohydrate	Fat
Very low-carb-appropriate	Classic ketogenic diet	0.8-1.4 g/kg/bw	Remainder	80%
Low-carb-appropriate	Can be ketogenic	0.8-2.8 g/kg/bw	Remainder	60-80%
Moderate-carb-appropriate	Not ketogenic	1.4-2.8 g/kg/bw	Remainder	30-60%
High-carb-appropriate	Not ketogenic	0.8-2.8 g/kg/bw	Remainder	Around 30%

Table 8. Macronutrient ratios of styles of Carb-Appropriate diet.

There is considerable variation in the macros for these diets. However, one thing remains constant—protein and fat intake should be set first, based on the needs of the individual, and then carbohydrate can be allocated from the remainder of calories.

SPECIFIC PROTEIN RECOMMENDATIONS

- Minimum RDA level: 0.8 g per kilogram of bodyweight (bw) per day
- For sports performance: 1.4-2 g per kg bw per day[255]
- If dieting hard or wanting to put on or retain maximal muscle: 2-2.8 g per kg bw per day[256] or more[257] (Figures ascertained from LBM amounts)

THE IMPORTANCE OF DIETARY FAT

Dietary fat is imperative for performance and an adequate dietary intake is essential for preserving hormonal status particularly for the sex-hormones (preservation), catabolic hormones like cortisol (reducing and/or modulating) and on overreaching-overtraining status. It has been suggested that at least 30% of calories should come from fats,[258] and this amount should be higher in low-carb and very low-carb diets in which more fuel is going to be derived from fatty acids than carbohydrate.

HIGHER 'CARB-APPROPRIATE'

Some people do respond fantastically well to Carb-Appropriate diets that include significant amounts of carbohydrate. I think this is one of the reasons we see some vegan and vegetarian advocates doing incredibly well on amounts of grains, fruit and legumes that would be inappropriate for some of us. Should they change? In short—No! If it ain't broke, don't fix it.

With a higher-carb variation on Carb-Appropriate nutrition, we need to ensure two requirements are met with respect to macronutrients: 1) That ample protein is consumed relative to your goals and 2) that ample fat is consumed to preserve optimal hormonal status.

HIGHER CARB-APPROPRIATE RECOMMENDATIONS

Fat: 30% or more of calories[258]

Protein: Between 1.4 g and 2.8 g or more, of protein per kilo of bodyweight per day.

Carbohydrate: The remainder of your daily calorie allotment (after fat and protein are removed from daily calories)

Best used for: Muscle gain, sports performance, general health IF highly tolerant to carbohydrates.

LOW-CARB DIETS

There is no universally accepted definition of a low-carbohydrate diet (LCD) and so it can be very confusing for the public (and researchers) to know exactly what is being spoken about when people use terms like 'LCHF' and low-carb.

It has been suggested that LCDs contain between 20 and 60 g of carbohydrate (typically less than 20% of total calories),[259] but it's also been suggested that anything up to 200 g of carbohydrate is 'low-carb'![260] For 'fat-adaptation' to occur optimally Westman and colleagues suggest that an LCD contains between 50 and 150 g of carbohydrate (but that this level may still not result in a level of 'nutritional ketosis').[260]

Confused yet?!

A meta-analysis of low-carbohydrate diets by Hu and colleagues in the American Journal of Epidemiology included a broader range of studies; including as 'low-carbohydrate' diets any that contained less than 45% of daily calories from carbohydrate.[261] This wholly unsatisfactory definition means that any diet containing less than the commonly recommended carbohydrate intake is by nature a low carbohydrate one. A more thorough definition is provided within a systematic review by Wheeler and colleagues in *Diabetes Care* which categorise LCDs as such[19]:

- very-low-carbohydrate diet: 21–70 g/day of carbohydrate

- moderately low–carbohydrate diet: 30 to <40% of kcal as carbohydrate
- moderate-carbohydrate diet: 40–65% of kcal as carbohydrate
- high-carbohydrate diet: >65% of kcal as carbohydrate

The lack of a definitive universally accepted definition for very low carbohydrate and low carbohydrate diets provides significant challenges to researchers seeking to synthesise and analyse the data, due to a lack of homogeneity between and within studies.[262] This causes confusion when evaluating the evidence for-and-against the use of low-carbohydrate diets when compared to standard best-practice diet guidelines.

But we can be clear on one point at least; that lowered-carb, moderate-to-high protein and moderate-to-high fat diets offer significant advantages for many people for satiety, compliance, body-fat loss, retention of muscle and a host of health conditions.

GENERAL LOW-CARB-APPROPRIATE RECOMMENDATIONS

Fat: 60-80% of calories

Protein: Between 1.4 g and 2.8 g or more, of protein per kilo of bodyweight per day

Carbohydrate: The remainder of your daily calorie allotment (after fat and protein are removed from daily calories)

Best used for: Weight-loss and weight maintenance. Can be appropriate for muscle gain and retention and is one of the better options for those suffering metabolic disorders.

If seeking help for a medical condition, see a suitably qualified health practitioner.

VERY LOW-CARB, KETOGENIC DIETS (VLCKDS)

Ketogenic diets are those that elicit the state of 'ketosis'. Ketosis refers to the production of ketone bodies, derived from fats (and some amino acids) for use as an alternative fuel in times of fasting or drastic carbohydrate restriction. A restriction of carbohydrate, either by fasting or by restricting dietary carbohydrate results in reduced insulin levels, thereby reducing lipogenesis (the creation of fats) and fat accumulation. When glycogen reserves become insufficient to supply the glucose necessary for normal fat oxidation (via the provision of oxaloacetate in the Krebs cycle) and for the supply of glucose to the Central Nervous System (CNS), an alternative fuel source is needed. CNS typically cannot utilise fat for fuel, as the common dietary lipids (long chain fatty acids) are almost always bound to albumin and are unable in this state to cross the blood-brain barrier. Fatty acids can desorp from albumin though,[263] and there are other subtle reasons why neurons, astrocytes and ganglia are more adapted to using glucose for fuel. Namely, that ßoxidation of fatty acids (FAs) demands more oxygen than the oxidation of glucose, thereby increasing the risk of hypoxia of neurons. Oxidation of FAs generates superoxide, causing increased oxidative stress for neurons, the rate of ATP generation from fatty acids (as compared to glucose) is slower, and so in times of rapid neuronal firing there is reduced fuel provision if FAs are the primary energy source for the brain.[264] This suggests an evolutionary-adaptive advantage to lowering the fatty oxidative capacity of brain cell mitochondria to avoid these challenges, and thus favours glucose oxidation in the brain.

Some dietary fats (such as short and medium chain triglycerides) are able to easily cross the blood-brain barrier (as they are not bound to albumin) and can be used extensively by neurons, but their availability is scarce in the typical diet and so the CNS relies primarily on glucose for fuel.

Alternative fatty acid derived fuels—the 'ketones' acetoacetate and ß-hydroxybutyric acid (BOHB) and acetone, do not promote the same raft of problems associated with LCFA metabolism in the brain.[264]

Ketone bodies are produced through a process called 'ketogenesis' in the liver to accommodate fuel demands during times of carbohydrate scarcity. Acetoacetate is the primary ketone body, with BOHB providing the primary circulating ketone. Technically BOHB is not a ketone body (as the ketone moiety has been reduced to a hydroxyl group) however, it functions as a primary fuel in the process of ketosis. Some Acetoacetate is produced under normal dietary conditions (which include moderate to high levels of carbohydrate) but this small amount is metabolised readily and rapidly by skeletal and heart tissue, resulting in only minimal levels of circulating ketones. It has been clinically observed that higher fat, moderated carbohydrate diets such as 'Paleo' and 'Primal' diets, also result in consistently higher levels of circulating BOHB than would be seen in standard western-style (higher-carbohydrate) diets. We would consider these diets to, therefore, be generally fat-adaptive, even when not very-low carbohydrate, but a dearth of evidence in this area requires further research.

When Acetoacetate is produced in large amounts, it is able to accumulate and be converted into the other ketone bodies (acetone and BOHB) leading to the presence of ketones in the blood and urine (ketonaemia and ketonuria respectively) and in the breath.

Ketones are utilised by tissue as a source of energy. BOHB results in two molecules of acetyl CoA which enter the Krebs cycle. In ketosis blood glucose levels stay within normal physiological limits due to the creation of glucose from glucogenic amino acids and via the liberation of glycerol during fatty oxidation.[i] All these factors of ketone, fatty-acid and glucose regulation are crucially important as

_____

[i] In silico models further suggest a plausible conversion of fatty acids to glucose 265. Kaleta, C., et al., *In Silico Evidence for Gluconeogenesis from Fatty Acids in Humans.* PLoS Computational Biology, 2011. **7**(7): p. e1002116., more likely to occur in periods of carbohydrate restriction.

certain cell types—in particular red blood cells (RBCs), lacking mitochondria, are only able to use glucose as a fuel source and thus the preservation of stable glucose levels is critical for survival.

KETOGENIC DIETS

The ketogenic diet itself is a form of LCHF diet that is very low in carbohydrate, low to moderate in protein and high in fat. It is often termed a 'very low carbohydrate ketogenic diet' (VLCKD). VLCKDs are characterised by the expression of ketone bodies in the blood, breath and urine. This expression of ketones is a 'functional' nutritional ketosis.

VLCKDs have been used to successfully treat childhood epilepsy since the 1920s with much of the scientific literature on the induction of ketosis and tolerability of the diet from this area. Systematic reviews and meta-analyses of the data conclude efficacy for the reduction of seizure frequency and severity.[266-270] Carbohydrate dose appears to be inversely proportionate to seizure activity in ketogenic diets, but with higher carbohydrate allowances in the diet increasing tolerability.[271, 272]

Macronutrient ratios of differing amounts have been shown to affect the ability of the body to reach a state nutritional ketosis.

A 'ketogenic ratio' of 4-parts fat to 1-part protein and carbohydrate (a '4:1 protocol') has been suggested as the best way to induce ketosis. This protocol forms the basis of the Johns Hopkins protocol[273] and is used by many medical practitioners and the research hospital of the same name in their treatment of childhood epilepsy. This ratio equates to approximately 80% of calories in the diet from fat. However, lower fat diets (with approximately 60%-75% of calories from fat) can induce ketosis effectively if a significantly high proportion of Medium Chain Triglycerides (MCTs) are included[274] and that these 'MCT diets' are also effective in the treatment of epilepsy and seizures.[275]

Huttenlocher demonstrated that a modified ketogenic diet with 60% of calories from MCTs and three-times more carbohydrate (18% vs. 6%), and ~50% more protein than a standard ketogenic diet could induce functional ketosis for epilepsy treatment.[276]

IS NUTRITIONAL KETOSIS SAFE?

Individual results to different diets will vary and a ketogenic diet may not apply to everyone, but nutritional ketosis is considered to be safe by most researchers in the field.

Ketosis elicited by dietary intervention has been described variously as 'functional ketosis'[277] or more commonly 'nutritional ketosis'. It has been claimed that Jeff Volek and Stephen Phinney coined the term 'nutritional ketosis' however the term can be found in the medical and scientific literature pre-dating Drs Volek and Phinney, for example in the work of Sargent and colleagues.[278] However, in many of the earlier texts ketosis, even if nutritionally induced (i.e. absent pathological aetiology) is considered to be a disadvantaged or dangerous state.

As early as 1960 Hans Krebs began to elucidate some of the mechanisms of interdependence between fatty acid and carbohydrate metabolism (for instance the effects on fatty acid metabolism and ketone production of reductions in oxaloacetate).[279] This began to differentiate the state of nutritional ketosis from disorders such as diabetic ketoacidosis (DKA). In 1966, Krebs differentiated 'physiologic' ketosis from pathological ketosis.[280]

Leading researchers in the LCHF field Jeff Volek and Stephen Phinney, consider the ten-fold physiologic range between 0.5 mmol/L or greater of BOHB to 5 mmol/L as the functional definition for 'nutritional ketosis'.[281, 282]

Ketoacidosis may also occur in the alcoholic. In alcoholic ketoacidosis gluconeogenesis is inhibited, creating an 'energy crisis', requiring increased fatty acid metabolism and ketone body formation.

Ketonaemia and nutritional ketosis resulting from ketogenic diets have been demonstrated to be safe when used in the treatment of epilepsy,[283-287] infantile spasms,[288] spinal cord injury,[289] and cancer.[290-292] Serious side effects have not been noted during studies for ketogenic diets and obesity,[78] hyperlipidaemia and diabetes, [293, 294] and they are safe for cardiovascular disease treatment.[88, 295]

NUTRITIONAL KETOSIS IS NOT KETOACIDOSIS

We are taught in under-grad University courses that ketosis is 'dangerous' because it is (wrongly) considered to be metabolic ketoacidosis. Diabetic ketoacidosis (DKA) is a potentially fatal condition characterised by a triad of hyperglycaemia (high blood-sugar levels), drastically increased total body ketone concentration and metabolic acidosis.[296] It results from uncontrolled diabetes mellitus and an inability of peripheral tissue to uptake glucose effectively, NOT from normal, nutritional ketosis.

A functional, nutritional ketosis (one absent of pathology) on the other hand is an adaptive response allowing the utilization of ketone bodies (in particular BOHB) by neurons and other tissue and reducing the need for carbohydrate (glucose) as a primary fuel in periods of carbohydrate scarcity. It has been demonstrated that insulin induced hypoglycaemic coma can be reversed by intravenous administration of BOHB,[297] BOHB effectively replaces glucose as fuel for neurons during starvation,[298] and preserves synaptic function even in the presence of glucose deprivation.[299]

CLINICAL APPLICATIONS OF LOW-CARB AND KETOGENIC DIETS

As mentioned earlier in this chapter VLCKDs have been used to successfully treat childhood epilepsy since the 1920s.[266, 267, 270] A 2012 Cochrane Database review of four randomised controlled trials, along with seven prospective

[136]

and four retrospective studies found ketogenic diets to be comparable to medication for the treatment of epilepsy.[268]

NEURODEGENERATIVE DISORDERS

High carbohydrate diets are hypothesised to play a role in the causation of Alzheimer's Disease (AD).[300]

A feasibility trial of five participants found reduced Parkinson's Disease (PD) activity after use of a ketogenic diet, which was tolerable and found suitable for the participants. Placebo effects cannot be ruled out as the trial was uncontrolled.[301] Positive effects from higher-fat diets may result wholly or partially from a greater intake of PUFAs in a diet inherently higher in total fat. In the Rotterdam Study, (a prospective cohort of 5289 people age greater or equal to 55 years) 51 participants with PD were identified. Intakes of MUFAs, PUFAs and total fat were correlated with lower risk of PD, with no association shown for cholesterol, saturated or trans-fats.[302]

OBESITY

Current dietary recommendations for obesity are centred on strategies that promote a lower calorie intake to reduce weight. The position statement on low-carbohydrate diets by Dietitians NZ states: "Dietitians New Zealand also considers there not to be any evidence that a diet high in fat and low in carbohydrates is more beneficial for sustained weight loss than any other dietary regimen that results in a lower intake of kilojoules."[303] This statement according to the first law of thermodynamics cannot be disputed but the roles of satiety, taste and potential metabolic advantages of diets varying in macronutrient content are not recognised in a simplistic 'calories in vs. calories out' proposition. It is highly likely that metabolic efficiencies and inefficiencies of various diets contribute to a metabolic advantage for weight loss.[23] It has been demonstrated that LCHF diets are more effective for early weight-loss than a standard low-fat, high-carbohydrate protocol[304-307] and that ad-libitum LCHF diets are as effective for weight control as calorie-restricted low-fat diets.[308] This may be due to an auto-regulation of energy intake due to the greater satiating effect of fats and protein, compared to carbohydrate.

Shai and colleagues investigated weight loss and cardiometabolic markers in people on either an energy restricted low-fat regime, energy restricted Mediterranean regime, or an unlimited energy low-carbohydrate regime. After 24 months, the low-carbohydrate regime had produced the greatest overall weight loss compared to the other two regimes, with more favourable changes to cardiometabolic markers including HDL cholesterol, triglycerides, and ratio of total cholesterol to HDL cholesterol.[84] Notwithstanding that effects observed *are* due to caloric restriction or caloric expenditure, the key point is that improved satiety, satisfaction, exercise expenditure and increased metabolic use of fuel occur automatically on lower-carbohydrate diets. In other words, these things do not need to be forced. This is amply demonstrated by the results seen in ad libitum vs. energy-restricted diets irrespective of a post-hoc analysis of calories consumed.

DIABETES

Obesity is closely linked with diabetes (type 2). Reduced bodyweight, BMI, blood glucose, total cholesterol, LDL cholesterol, triglycerides and urea levels were reduced in 64 patients following a ketogenic diet for 56 weeks with a significant increase in HDL (P<0.0001).[309]

A controlled trial by Hussain and colleagues compared over 24 weeks the effect of a low calorie (2200 calorie) 'best-practice' diet with a low-carbohydrate, ad libitum, ketogenic diet in both diabetic and non-diabetic participants. There were significant reductions in weight, BMI, waist circumference, glycated haemoglobin in both diabetics and non-diabetics following a VLCKD versus a low-calorie diet. Interestingly blood lipid profiles were improved for TAG, LDL and total cholesterol (all reduced), and HDL (increased) significantly only in the VLCKD group (D2 and ND) with some worsening in those following a low-calorie diet. Also significant—there was noted a *worsening* of total cholesterol and triglycerides in non-diabetics following a standard calorie-restricted diet.[310]

A 44 month follow up of 16 diabetic patients following a low-carbohydrate diet (50% fat, 20% carbohydrate, 30% protein) showed statistically significant (P<0.001) improvements in weight, BMI, HbA1C, HDL-C and HDL to total cholesterol ratio.[311]

[139]

CANCER

Cancer cells are predominantly glycolytic. The shift from normal aerobic metabolism to glycolysis in cancer cells is known as the 'Warburg Effect' as described by Otto Warburg.[312] Mutations and further growth in tumours are related to disturbed energy metabolism, and due to the reliance on higher carbohydrate diets in dietary guidelines for health, some standards of current care may contribute to the progression of tumours. On the other hand, calorie restricted or ketogenic diets may be effective to reduce these metabolic maladies.[313]

Reviews of the published literature for both animal and human studies suggest a role in cancer treatment for the ketogenic diet as it may be 'toxic' to cancer cells and effectively starves them of priority fuel for continued growth and progression, and is well tolerated and safe for patients.[314, 315]

AUTISM

Very early (and highly speculative) preliminary evidence suggests a possible adjunct treatment role of a ketogenic diet in the reduction of seizures in autistic children[316] and more broadly in reducing symptoms of autism.[317]

MODIFIED MCT KETOGENIC DIET RECOMMENDATIONS

Fat: 60% or more of calories
Typically, high-MCT modified ketogenic protocols had almost the entire fat intake from MCTs, although we have found this to be unnecessary and simply focussing on using MCT containing

foods such as coconut oil and coconut cream or using MCT oils in food liberally is sufficient.

Protein: Between 1.4 g and 3 g of protein per kilo of bodyweight per day

Carbohydrate: The remainder of your daily calorie allotment (after fat and protein are removed from daily calories)

CLASSIC KETOGENIC DIET RECOMMENDATIONS

Fat: 80% of calories

Protein: Between 1.2 g and 3 g of protein per kilo of bodyweight per day

Carbohydrate: The remainder of your daily calorie allotment (after fat and protein are removed from daily calories)

Best used for: Aggressive weight-loss, weight-maintenance, cognitive benefits, improved satiety, treatment for a host of disorders under the care of a suitably qualified practitioner

CHAPTER 11

PUTTING IT TOGETHER

Getting more specific with Carbohydrate Appropriate nutrition

The following pages contain specific information on what you can start to do right now to begin to eat (and live!) more Carb-Appropriate. Use these tips and strategies as a guideline and adjust to fit your needs. As always if you have specific concerns, health conditions or are using medications consult a suitably qualified health practitioner. See the website of the Holistic Performance Institute for HPN™ Certified Practitioners www.hpn.ac.nz

RECOMMENDED SUPPLEMENTS

- Fish or krill oil (or flax oil or vegan, algal-derived DHA/EPA)
- A multi-nutrient formula
- Protein powder

Note: I am a co-founder of the NuZest company and so I recommend Good Green Stuff *as a multi-nutrient product and* Clean Lean Protein *as a protein supplement. However, there are many good brands that can fit the bill for you.*

HYDRATION

You should aim for at least two litres of water per day with an additional litre taken per hour of training. If training for two hours or longer also take 500-1000 mg of sodium (per litre) with your water.

MORNING HYDRATION RITUAL

- ½ squeezed lemon in 1 large glass of water, fish oils (see dosing guide)
- In 1 large glass of water: 1 tsp *Good Green Stuff* or other quality multi-nutrient formula.

Continue to drink water frequently and liberally, according to taste and desire throughout the day.

EAT 9 CUPS OF VEGETABLES & BERRIES PER DAY

- 3 cups of dark green, leafy vegetables
- 3 cups red, orange, blue or purple vegetables or berries
- 3 cups of sulphur-rich vegetables (cauliflower, broccoli, asparagus, Brussels sprouts, turnips, onions, garlic)

Eat most	Eat according to carb tolerance	Avoid
Full-fat containing meat, poultry, fish Free-range eggs Full-fat dairy products Green vegetables Orange, yellow and red vegetables (capsicums, peppers and tomatoes and pumpkin) Olive, flax, hempseed and coconut oils Nuts and seeds Avocado Berries Fermented vegetables (sauerkraut, kimchi)	Kumara, yams Whole, unprocessed grains (e.g. quinoa, millet, amaranth) Legumes (e.g. lentils, mung beans) Sprouted are preferred	All sugars and substitutes Bread, pasta, cookies, crackers and other bakery goods All 'low-fat' products Common vegetable oils (safflower, sunflower, corn, soy)
Green, white and herbal teas liberally Up to 1 x alcoholic drink per day for men and 1 drink every second day for women	Small amounts of coffee OK (Up to 3 x black [or with small amounts cream or full-fat milk] coffees per day before 2 pm) Low sugar (under 3g per 100 ml) kombucha and coconut kefir – up to 200 ml per day	Sodas Fruit juice

Table 9: Carb-Appropriate sample food list

[145]

Approximate Quantities Per Meal			
Protein Foods 1-2 palm sized portions	*Healthy Fats* Approx. 1 tsp. per 20 kg bodyweight	*Vegetables* (3 fist-sized servings at lunch and dinner)	*Additions*
Beef (free range) Chicken (free range) Fish (wild) Pork (free range) Occasionally: Tempeh or Tofu 2 x fist sized portions of sprouted legumes as a vegetarian protein option	Added to food: Avocado (0-60 kg ½ - over 60 kg whole) Olive Oil Hempseed Oil Used for cooking: Ghee (clarified butter) Coconut Oil/Cream	Beet greens, asparagus, bok choy, borage, broccoli, Brussels sprouts, cabbage, celery, chickweed, chicory, cress, dandelion leaves, endive, rocket (arugula), kale, lettuces, pak choy, spinach, sprouted lentils, mung bean sprouts, radish greens, carrot greens, radishes, Swiss chard, turnip greens	Feel free to use a fist sized portion of: Kumara, yams, parsnip or 'ancient grains' (quinoa, millet, wild rice) to meals. 1-2 pieces of fruit may also be added if you have reached goal weight/body-fat level. Berries and berry powders can be liberally added to any meal. Carrot and pumpkin can be added to meals in small amounts.
1 x egg per 20 kg of bodyweight as a protein option			

Table 10. Approximate quantities of foods in a Carb-Appropriate meal plan.

Example Daily Menu Plan (70 kg ~ Fat Loss Goal)		
On rising	½ squeezed lemon in 1 large glass of water	3 x 1000 mg fish oil caps
7 AM	3 x eggs with kumara mash or hash, spinach and a small (1/4) serve avocado OR ½ cup of low-grain muesli or granola with additional berries and a little full-fat milk or cream of your choice	
12 PM	2 x fist sized portions of sprouted lentils and mung beans with mixed green salad, a sprinkling of pumpkin seeds with ½ avocado dressed with a little rock salt and pepper	
4 PM	Smoothie: 2 x scoops *Clean Lean Protein*, 1 tsp. *Blackcurrant powder*, 2 tsp. (1 scoops) *Good Green Stuff*, ½ cup frozen berries, 1 Tbsp. Hempseed oil	
7 PM or later	1 x palm sized portion of grass feed, free range steak with 3 x fist-sized portions of mixed rocket, spinach and grated carrot. 1 Tbsp. of olive oil, mixed with lemon juice and salt/pepper as dressing. Add kumara, yams, pumpkin as desired.	3 x 1000 mg fish oil caps

Table 11. Sample menu for a Carb-Appropriate nutrition plan.

CARB-APPROPRIATE STRATEGIES

DON'T GO SHOPPING ON AN EMPTY STOMACH

Go shopping after a meal…not before. We all know what can happen when we go to the supermarket starving—we buy crap. Shopping when satisfied will drive better food choices.

MAKE TOO MUCH FOR DINNER SO THAT YOU HAVE LUNCH FOR THE FOLLOWING DAY

This is my top strategy for compliance. Lunch can so often be the meal that derails our efforts. It can be difficult to find a quality lunch option, and if we get to the point of genuine hunger and are faced with other not-so-good options, we're likely to take them. By making too much dinner and putting aside lunch for the following day, we ensure that we have a great quality meal and it saves us a lot of time and money!

USE SMOOTHIES

Smoothies are a god-send for when you need a simple, effective, nutrient-dense meal and have little time to prepare.

Your smoothie should include:

Protein + vegetables + berries + a healthy fat

Here's my favourite smoothie recipe:

- 3 x scoops *Clean Lean Protein*
- ½ cup blueberries
- 2 x Tbsp. peanut butter

- A splash of olive and hempseed oil
- 1-3 cups of mixed green vegetables (kale, spinach, puha, dandelion, etc.)

Additionally, I may add a piece of fruit and/or creatine or other supplements if trying to achieve a particular goal (muscle gain or increased strength and power).

CREATE A 'BLOCK' TO NEGATIVE EATING (ESP. AFTER WORK)

One of the worst times for habitual, mindless eating is immediately after work. We get home tired, sometimes hungry (especially if we are not yet that well fat-adapted) and reach for sugary treats…or in fact, anything!

A great way to 'block' this behaviour is to simply tell yourself that you must have a different food choice before you have a treat. I have had great success with clients by having them eat a salad as soon as they get home. This serves several purposes. 1) They eat more veggies! 2) The veggies taste better (because they are hungry!). 3) They are more satiated and less likely to snack after the salad. 4) It provides a behavioural 'block' that changes the pattern of eating mindlessly immediately after work.

USE HERBAL TEA TO CURB SUGAR CRAVINGS AT NIGHT

Like the tip before, this strategy is a behavioural 'block' that changes a pattern of overeating at night. Often the night time cravings are very patterned and habitual, and may have less basis in pure physiology. By having a cup of tea when we begin to crave we are able to reduce the craving. Often this also serves as a signal to the body-mind complex to relax, reset and chill and this can have positive effects on sleep too.

CHAPTER 12

THE OTHER STUFF

Lifestyle, movement, sleep, stress and mindfulness

Achieving any physical or mental goal involves so much more than diet alone. Whether improved performance on the field, in the ring or on the platform, or improving mental and cognitive ability, or simply looking and feeling better, diet is just one part of the picture of total health and performance.

Our patterns of behaviour are drastically affected by stress, our bodies are directly affected by stress and a plethora of mind-body interrelationships (including the obvious—movement and exercise) affect how well our body can function and how it responds to nutrients. Any nutrition book would be remiss to not mention these factors. And while a full evaluation of these is beyond the scope of *this* book (hint…) it is important to incorporate more than just nutrition strategies into your life if you are to achieve optimal results.

SLEEP

It's probably fair to say that many of us either don't get either sleep or the *quality of sleep* that we require to perform at our best. In fact, most of the people I see in practice have some combination of trouble getting to sleep, fitful or restless sleep, short sleep duration (early waking, without being able to get back to sleep), or they simply wake up feeling like crap!

There is no one-size-fits-all recommendation for sleep, and some of our 'best practice' guidelines are perhaps based more on a collective belief than evidence. It is clear however that sleep duration, and what is best for *you* is dependent on a number of different factors including genetics (some people may have genes and gene mutations causing shorter sleep duration),[318] activity (if you work or train intensely you need more sleep in order to recover) and the amount of latent mental activity (stress, over-activity of the mind etc.) that you exhibit due to your environment, career, family-life and personal disposition.

According to the National Sleep Foundation of the US, which convened an expert panel to evaluate optimal sleep times, the recommended amounts of sleep for various ages are[319]:

0-3 months: 14-17 hours per night

4-11 months: 12-15 hours

1-2 years: 11-14 hours

3-5 years: 10-13 hours

6-13 years: 9-11 hours

14-17 years: 8-10 hours

18-64 years: 7-9 hours

65+ years: 7-8 hours

So most of us should really be aiming to get at least seven hours of good quality sleep per day/night. If we exercise or are highly active in our work, or in a high stress environment our needs are likely to be greater.

WHAT HAPPENS IF WE DON'T GET ENOUGH SLEEP? At its most extreme sleep-deprivation is fatal. Lab rats when denied sleep completely, die within two to three weeks. The brain's ability to function deteriorates markedly as a consequence of too little sleep. Speech may slur, cognition decreases and thought patterning becomes more rigid. It's as if the brain, if not given sufficient rest goes into an 'auto-pilot' mode and has much more trouble with creativity, problem-solving and troubleshooting in ways that require lateral and non-linear thinking.

Emotional disturbances result from sleep deprivation too. The transient anxiety and irritability we all feel from the odd late night can develop into more serious anxiety and depressive disorders with prolonged sleep deprivation.

Physical performance drops in response to inadequate sleep. Endurance and strength levels begin to drop, ocular function deteriorates, fine motor control and co-ordination deteriorate and glucose metabolism is less efficient.

Some of the more common reasons for the lack of sleep quantity and quality are shift work, caffeine, nicotine, alcohol, a poor diet, and emotional stress. Luckily these are all things that we can deal with.

TEN SIMPLE STEPS TO A BETTER SLEEP

ASK YOURSELF: "WHY AM I HAVING TROUBLE SLEEPING?" (AKA 'HOW IS THIS SERVING ME?')

Rather than just launching into 'treatments' for insomnia, we are much better served by looking at the reasons why we don't sleep well.

We have many, many things on our minds, from work, relationship or other 'stressors'. However, contrary to what we may think, it isn't the 'stressor' that stresses us out…It is our relationship to it.

While removing stressful situations from our lives (or more commonly removing ourselves from them) can drastically improve our overall stress picture, if we simply remove stressors, without recognising *why* they stress us out, we may soon find other situations arising that provide stress for the same underlying reasons.

Usually, our stress-driven relationships with these situations result from aspects of security, self-worth, loss or attachment. Consulting a practitioner who can help release self-limiting beliefs and behaviours can help ensure a better night sleep, but also just being aware of them, and being more mindful can also bring great rewards.

[154]

CREATE A RITUAL

Sometimes we continue in our 'work-day' mind-set even when we are at home. We haven't really disengaged from our day and provided a signal to our body-mind complex to go into relaxation mode. Creating a ritual helps to do this. It is a somatic and psychological signal that it is now time to stop thinking and worrying about the concerns of the day and instead to relax into rest and recovery.

This is one of the reasons I often counsel my clients to do a short meditation when they first get home. It provides a 'bookend' to the working day and can really help you to settle into a much more relaxed state. Other great rituals include breathing exercises, yoga, whole brain exercises, and one of my favourites—making a cup of relaxing herbal tea. (Peppermint, chamomile, valerian, passionflower and skullcap are all relaxing herbs - check with your Naturopath or Medical Herbalist to see what is best for you.)

TURN THE DAMN TV OFF AND DON'T STAY ON THE COMPUTER TOO LATE!

Our daily rhythms are heavily affected by light intensity. In a natural state as light intensity drops (when the sun goes down) we begin to change our balance of hormonal biochemistry to the relaxing and sleep inducing hormones rather than the stimulatory hormones, epinephrine and norepinephrine.

TV and computer screens emit a high light intensity that can practically fool the brain/body into awakening, and the heavily stimulatory themes on TV add to this effect.

I have seen profound results in clients sleep quality when they stop watching TV before 9 pm and *remove the television from the bed room!*

(Note: The bedroom should be a place for sleeping, reading, relaxing and having sex only!) However, in the interests of full-disclosure, I must confess that I have recently purchased a TV for my bedroom! NetFlix and chill…

READ FICTION

Reading fiction seems to do wonders for relaxing the mind and helping sleep. While non-fiction can cause us to begin to plan and project into the future (potentially driving a moderate stress response) fiction seems to do the opposite.

Heavily violent or disturbing themes may do the opposite though so be aware of what works best for you.

HAVE A BATH

A warm bath or shower is relaxing in and of itself, but the primary sleep benefit of taking a bath or shower before bed is the *drop in temperature* that occurs afterwards. This drop in temperature is another signal from the environment that the day is ending and this further increases the release of relaxing hormones (especially melatonin). Of course, you can get fancy, add some relaxing essential oils, put on some

Barry Manilow or whatever else floats your boat too…Hey, whatever you do in your bath is your own business!

MEDITATE

The constant buzzing and whirring of the mind are perhaps the biggest obstacle to sleep. Many people try in vain to 'switch the mind off'. This is an exercise in futility and, in my opinion, a devaluing of the wonderful properties of the mind. It is, after all, a wonderful thought producing machine! Why would you want to stop the mind doing what it does?

But we can find some 'middle ground' and simply let thoughts *be* and not repress them nor get carried away with them—either of which provides energy to the thoughts, promoting and sustaining them, and this prevents us from sleeping.

Using contemplative exercises such as *mindfulness of breath* can allow us to become calmer and we can begin, in time, to simply let thoughts arise and fall without the attachment that drives further thought-processing and stress.

(For tips on meditation see: *Time Rich Cash Optional: an unconventional guide to happiness*)

DON'T TAKE YOUR WORK HOME

Leave your work at the office.

If you bring it home, there is even more of an imperative to resume unfinished tasks, and even the mere sight of it can drive subconscious processes associated with adrenal stress response. By leaving it at the office, you have both 'out of sight, out of mind' and you have created a clear delineation between work time-space and home time-space.

USE HERBAL MEDICATIONS OR SUPPLEMENTS

Try some gentle herbs and supplements. The herbs already suggested can be gentle aids to a better sleep. Other nutritional supplements (especially magnesium and melatonin[i]) may also be useful for many people.

See a Clinical Nutritionist or Naturopath for advice on what would work best for you.

AVOID CAFFEINE AND ALCOHOL BEFORE BED

This is a complete no-brainer! Caffeine is obviously a stimulant, and even if you don't think that late cup o' Joe is affecting your ability to sleep, or your quality of sleep, it is in all likelihood providing for a more restless slumber. Avoid caffeine for at least 6 hours before bed. Many of my clients report that at least 9 hours is best.

Alcohol also affects the quality of sleep. Although we get to sleep more easily as a result of a wee tipple we are less able to enter the deepest states of sleep if we have over-imbibed. I know that if I have a few wines too close to bed-time, it's a sure-bet that my sleep will be less effective and more restless.

---

[i] Melatonin is a restricted medicine in New Zealand

WATCH OUT FOR THOSE MEDICATIONS!

Many medications can interfere with sleep patterns including asthma relief medications (as they are stimulatory to the CNS), pseudoephedrine containing cough and cold remedies and antidepressants. If you think your medications are affecting your sleep talk with your health provider about ways to limit the effect they may be having (but try to avoid sleeping pills, they don't give a good quality of sleep and are prone to the development of dependency.)

DON'T EAT TOO MUCH BEFORE BED

Eating too much before bed can upset digestive processes. Whether this occurs and to what extent is both highly individual and can be dependent on what you eat. If, after following the other recommendations in this book, you are still experiencing a poor sleep, and especially if you feel 'gripey' or have any pain, discomfort or bloating during the night or on arising, try reducing your food before bed. Eat your last meal about three hours before bed and be aware of any foods that you may be intolerant to.

RECOMMENDATIONS:

- Sleep: 6.5-9 hours per night
- If you are woken up by your alarm more than one or two nights per week you are either not sleeping long enough or your sleep is too disturbed to be properly restful

- Train: Move daily — whether it is a walk, jog, weights session or yoga. Simply do something daily!
- Also, do at least two heavy weight training or weight-bearing exercise sessions per week

MINDFULNESS

"Put simply mindfulness is seeing things for what they are. It is being open to what is going on around you, without attachment and without reaction.

It is developing the 'watcher' or the 'observer' within. Our minds are perpetual motion machines that create thought after thought. Mindfulness is recognising that these thoughts are transient and these thoughts are not us.

By observing our thoughts and emotions, by developing the 'watcher' within, we can see that our thoughts are not us. There is something deeper than this. We know this simply because we can become mindful, we can 'watch' our thoughts and emotions arise…and so we know that they are things that happen, and are in fact things that we 'do' and cannot, therefore, be 'us'."

~ Cliff (from Choosing You!*)*

Mindfulness is key to being able to institute new patterns of behaviour that lead to lasting change. Try a mindfulness of breath meditation every morning and possibly every evening. Yoga is also a great way to get your movement and meditation in one hit.

There are several ways that you can encourage mindfulness in your life. I strongly recommend you put some time (as little as 10 min) each and every day into one mindfulness activity. You can do the same activity every day at the same time, at different times or perform different activities as you feel like it. An activity that suits one person will not suit everyone. Be a power unto yourself...the main thing is that you do it!

I try to do a sitting meditation for at least 20 min every day, usually first thing in the morning and additionally at night. I find that doing this allows me to be calmer, more focussed and more 'centred' during the day by encouraging greater mindfulness of what is going on in and around me.

Doing it in the morning, before anything else, also makes certain that I do it, don't forget to do it, or put it off as I become distracted by the other commitments of the day. Often I will do another 'mindful' activity during the day as well as a lying meditation before bed.

With meditation and mindfulness, there is no 'right way' to do it. There are no levels of achievement nor any sensations, thoughts, feelings or visions that you 'should' experience or feel. There are effective methods that can help you to be mindful but there is no right or wrong way. The time you spend meditating is time for you. Allow yourself the time to simply do what you are doing (be it sitting, lying or an activity).

Your mind WILL wander, that's what it has evolved to do, and it is completely fine and natural. With meditation and mindfulness, we are not trying to clear the mind of thoughts. In fact, what happens is actually inconsequential. The key is to do it! Simply be, return your focus gently to your activity and above all be kind to yourself.

There is no failure and no destination. The goal is in the doing.

As you can see any activity can be mindful…you just have to approach it, treat it and do it mindfully.

Perform at least one exercise mindfully each day…You may even notice that you are becoming more mindful during other tasks too.

For more information on goal-setting, meditation, mindfulness and finding your passion and life-purpose check out *Time Rich Practice*, *Time Rich Cash Optional* and *Choosing You!* By Cliff.

CHAPTER 13

MIC DROP

Can't we all just get along?

There is so much confusion on the topic of what a good diet actually *is*. And to be honest, we as practitioners, researchers, scientists and health coaches of any type or description need to take some of the blame for this.

We have polarised opinions by so strongly wanting to be 'right' that we have ended up blinding ourselves to the commonalities in great diets of all types.

There is no one BEST diet for everyone…

We are all fond of saying that there is no one-size-fits-all and yet in the same breath will debate the minutiae and fail to leave our own confirmation biases at the door. We are so addicted to wanting to be 'right' that our cognitive dissonance is preventing the public from receiving a truly pragmatic, holistic, evidence-based message of good quality nutrition.

Carb-Appropriate is a diet book.

Unashamedly…

Criticism may be levelled that it is a means to make money (it is) and that the diet advice it prescribes is just one of many means that could be effective (Yep—it's that too!) But I hope that people will see my work for what it is—an attempt to help people to better understand nutrition, the science behind it, and most importantly the application of it that works best *for them*.

Raw vegan, vegetarian, paleo, primal, clean-eating, low-sugar, no-sugar, high-protein, high-fat, low-carb, high-carb…ad infinitum, ad nauseum…all work at the right time and for the right person. The foundation for any diet that works though, for all people, almost all of the time, is one based on natural, whole and unprocessed foods. This is a naturalistic approach but it is one that is overwhelming based on scientific evidence (along with, if I can be so bold, *common sense*).

Is there *any* place for processed foods?

Yes!

But we don't have the same freedom to eat according to how we feel when eating foods that are packed with highly-processed carbohydrates, added sugar and high levels of trans- and omega-6 fats than if we simply were to eat as much natural food as we'd like.

In spite of the vigorous debate in the nutrition field, most of us are singing from the same song-sheet. Unfortunately, many academics and practitioners may fall victim to vilifying a particular nutrient or diet, or launch ad hominem attacks against other clinicians and scientists in the field. This can further confuse the public and while we are debating the science in our clinics and faculties they can be swayed towards getting advice and information from dubious sources.

I must admit that it is fun to debate the nuances of nutrition, but we shouldn't let that distract us from the end-game of encouraging better outcomes for public health and society (especially for those most at risk) by providing a clear, simple and effective message of healthy, wholefood-based nutrition.

I hope that the Carb-Appropriate method has helped you to understand more about a healthy diet and how you can use it to achieve your health and performance goals.

Blessings,

THE AUTHOR

CLIFF HARVEY

Cliff Harvey is a registered clinical nutritionist, naturopath, researcher, author and speaker. He is considered one of the leading practitioners in the area of fat metabolism and metabolic efficiency.

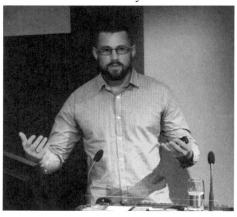 Cliff has been applying real-food, low- and lower-carbohydrate diets since 1998 and is one of the first, and certainly one of the longest-serving practitioners in the LCHF arena in Australasia. Over his nearly two decades in practice, he has helped thousands around the globe to live happier, healthier lives. He continues to inspire through his writing, speaking and clinical practice, and is involved in ongoing research in the area of metabolic adaptation to higher fat, lower carbohydrate diets with the Human Potential Centre at AUT University.

He is the founder of Holistic Performance Nutrition™ a post-tertiary college and continuing education body for practitioners, teaching evidence-based performance nutrition from the perspective of (holistic) clinical nutrition.

Cliff's practice is located in Auckland, New Zealand and he regularly travels the globe to teach.

More can be found at:

www.cliffharvey.com

www.hpn.ac.nz

For information on research results and upcoming studies follow HPN on Facebook:

www.facebook.com/HolisticPerformanceNutrition

GLOSSARY

Term or Abbreviation	Description
Acetyl CoA	Acetyl coenzyme A. An important molecule for energy production including balancing fatty acid, carbohydrate and ketone body metabolism.
Acidosis	Increased acidity in the blood (and other tissue).
Ad libitum	'As much as one desires'. Commonly used in nutrition research to indicate that a participant may eat as much (or as much of a certain food0 as they desire.
Aerobic	Requiring or using oxygen (usually as part of a metabolic process).
Aetiology	In medicine the study of the cause of disease. Also a noun for the causes of disease i.e. "The aetiology of the disease is unclear".
AI	Adequate intake. An approximate measure of nutrient intake within a population. Used when an RDA cannot be determined.
ADHD	Attention Deficit Hyperactivity Disorder.

Allopathic/Allopathy	A term used to describe the orthodox treatment of symptoms by drug ad surgical interventions.
Amino acid	A simple organic compound containing both a carboxyl ($-COOH$) and an amino ($-NH_2$) group. These function as the 'building blocks' of the proteins that make up cells, organs and tissue.
Androgen	A steroid hormone associated with male sex characteristics.
Androstenedione	A weak androgen and precursor of testosterone.
Antibiotic	A medical drug used to treat bacterial infections.
AMY1	The gene that codes for salivary amylase, the carbohydrate digesting enzyme in the mouth.
Asthma	An inflammatory respiratory condition often triggered by hypersensitivity or allergy.
Atherogenic	Tending towards the promotion of fatty deposits in arteries.
AUT	Auckland University of Technology
Autism	A mental condition usually present from childhood characterised by difficulty communicating and forming relationships with other

[169]

people and in using language and abstract concepts.

Autoimmunity — An immune response against the body's own cells.

Bifidobacteria — A common, plentiful genus of anaerobic bacteria found in the human gut.

BMI — Body Mass Index. A measure of height-to-weight that is used to estimate healthy weight ranges. This measure is complicated by increased muscle mass and so is not considered a good reference for athletic populations.

BOHB — Beta-hydroxybutyric acid. One of the major ketone (fuel) bodies.

Caesarean section — A surgical, non-vaginal method of delivering a baby.

Carb-Appropriate — A method for determining the carbohydrate requirement and tolerance of an individual for health and performance.

Calorie — A unit of energy. Equivalent to the energy required to raise one gram of water by one degree Celsius.

Campylobacter — A genus of commonly pathogenic bacteria causing gastroenteritis in humans.

Cardiometabolic	Concerning both the heart and metabolism especially in diseased states.
Cardioprotective	A substance or factor considered to be beneficial for cardiovascular health.
Cardiovascular	Concerning the heart and circulatory system.
Carotenoids	Organic pigments found in plants and some bacteria and fungi. In humans functioning as antioxidants and as pro-vitamin (A) compounds.
CD	Crohn's Disease – an IBD and autoimmune condition affecting the gut. It can express anywhere from the mouth to anus.
CDI	*Clostridium dificile* infection – A common cause of diarrhea and colitis.
Cholesterol	A sterol lipid used in the creation of various structural and functional compounds in the body including the steroid hormones (e.g. testosterone, cortisol, oestrogen).
Clostridium	A genus of pathogenic bacteria from the phylum *Firmicutes.*
Cochrane Review	Reviews of primary research in human health care and health policy. Internationally

	recognised as the highest standard of evidence-based health care.
Coeliac Disease	A chronic autoimmune disease affecting the gut wall, impeding nutrient digestion. Caused by a severe intolerance to gluten protein from grains such as wheat, barley and rye.
Cortisol	A steroid stress hormone that aids gluconeogenesis and the metabolism of fats, carbohydrates and proteins along with reducing immune function. It may reduce insulin sensitivity over the long-term.
DHA	Docosahexaenoic acid. Omega-3 fat found in krill and fish oil.
DHEA	Didehydroepiandrosterone (commonly dehydroepiandrostendione), a steroid hormone and intermediate converted to oestrogens and testosterone. Also a neurosteroid with its own biological activity.
Diabetes	A group of metabolic disorders characterized by high blood glucose levels.
DKA	Diabetic Ketoacidosis. A severe and potentially fatal

	condition of extremely high ketone levels and high blood glucose seen in uncontrolled diabetics. (Note: NOT Nutritional Ketosis. See 'Ketosis')
Dopamine	Tyrosine derived catecholamine hormone. Known as our 'reward' hormone and also involved in smooth muscle (and other) functions throughout the body.
Dysglycaemia	Abnormal blood-sugar levels.
E. coli	Escherichia coli. A common, usually non-pathogenic bacteria found in large amounts in the gut. Pathogenic strains can cause food poisoning.
Enterococcus	A genus of bacteria from the phylum *Firmicutes*, some of which are responsible for opportunistic infections.
Enteromammary	An immune-cell mediated pathway between the gut and the mammary glands. Allows for transmission of beneficial bacteria to the newborn.
EPA	Eicosapentaenoic acid. An omega-3 fatty acid found in fish and krill oil.

Epinephrine	One of our major 'fight-or-flight' stress hormones. (Also known as *adrenaline*).
Faecal calprotectin	A measure used to indicate intestinal inflammation (for example in diseases such as Crohn's Disease).
Fatty Acid (FA)	A carboxylic acid with a long aliphatic tail (chain). A component of triglycerides (with glycerol) or as free fatty acids (FFAs). A primary fuel source.
Genetic	Relating to genes or heredity.
GI	Glycaemic Index. A measure of the rise in blood sugar from ingesting 50g of carbohydrate from food. (Can also be in reference to Gastrointestinal).
Glucogenic	Something that encourages the creation of glucose within the body.
Gluconeogenesis	The creation (genesis) of new (neo) glucose from either glycerol from fat or from amino acids from protein.
Glycaemia	The presence of (or related to) glucose in the blood e.g. 'hypoglycaemia' or low blood sugar.
Glycation	When a sugar (glucose, fructose or galactose) binds without the action of an

	enzyme to a protein. This causes stiffening and damage to the protein resulting in dysfunction.
Glycerol	A simple sugar alcohol that forms the 'backbone' of triglycerides. Can be converted to glucose for use as fuel.
Glycolysis	The process of breaking down glucose (carbohydrate) for fuel.
Goitre	Swelling of the neck resulting from enlargement of the thyroid gland. Usually related to an iodine deficiency.
HbA1C	Glycated haemoglobin. The haemoglobin protein can be 'glycated' by glucose in the blood and thus provides a measure to indicate average blood glucose levels over time.
HCLF	High-carb, low-fat.
HDL	High-density lipoprotein. A protein carrier for cholesterol. Transports cholesterol back to the liver for processing from peripheral tissue.
Homo Sapiens	The genus and species name for modern man.

Hyperinsulinaemia	The presence of high (hyper-) levels of insulin in the blood (aemia).
Hyperlipidaemia	A term denoting high levels of one or a combination of cholesterol, lipoproteins or triglycerides in the blood.
Hypothesis	A proposed solution. Used as a starting point for further investigation.
In silico	Performed (studied or demonstrated) in a computer model.
In situ	Performed or studied in the original or natural position.
In vivo	Studied or demonstrated in a live, whole organism (such as a study performed in humans).
Insulin	The major storage hormone in the body. Promotes disposal of glucose and fatty acids into tissue and encourages retention of triglycerides in adipose (fat) tissue.
Ketogenic Diet (KD)	A high-fat, low-carbohydrate, low-to-moderate protein diet designed to induce 'nutritional ketosis'.
Ketone	In nutrition, this refers to 'ketone bodies' (acetone, acetoacetic acid, and beta-hydroxybutyric acid) —

	water-soluble molecules that are produced by the liver from fatty acids and some amino acids during periods of fasting or carbohydrate restriction.
Ketosis	The state of producing ketones for fuel. Indicated by the presence of ketones in the blood (ketonaemia) or urine (ketonuria). Also known as 'Nutritional Ketosis' (NK) and usually considered to be a blood BOHB reading of greater than 0.5 mmol/L.
Krill	Small crustaceans that are high in omega 3 oils commonly used in supplements.
Lactobacillus	A genus of ('good') bacteria found commonly in the body.
LCD	Low carbohydrate diet.
LCHF	Low-carb, high-fat.
LDL	Low-density lipoprotein. A protein carrier for cholesterol. Transports cholesterol to peripheral tissue and organs for use.
Leaky gut	A common term for increased intestinal permeability.
Lipid	Naturally occurring chemicals that include fats, waxes, sterols, fat-soluble vitamins (A, D, E, and K),

monoglycerides, diglycerides, triglycerides and phospholipids.

LPS
Lipopolysaccharide. An inflammatory endotoxin released from the membrane of certain bacteria.

MCT
Medium Chain Triglyceride. A triglyceride (fat) in which at least two of the three fatty acid chains are medium in length (chain length of between six and ten carbons).

Melatonin
One of the tryptophan derived hormones. A powerful antioxidant and involved in the initiation of the relaxation-sleep phase of our circadian cycle.

Meta-analysis
A statistical method for combing the results of studies to provide greater statistical power.

Metabolism
The changing of chemical structures within the body. Denotes all chemical processes occurring within a living organism.

Metabolic Typing
The categorization of people according to their supposed efficiency of use of the macronutrients. The 'Metabolic Typing Diet' has

	not been demonstrated to be effective.
Methylation	The addition of a methyl group to a molecule.
Microbiome	The collective genomes of the organisms that on or within the body.
Microbiota	The collective organisms that live on or within the body.
Mineral (essential)	In nutrition a solid, naturally occurring, inorganic substance essential for life.
Mitochondria	The cell's 'powerhouse' responsible for aerobic energy production.
Morbidity	A diseased state or symptom.
Mortality	Death.
MUFA	Monounsaturated fatty acid. A fatty acid with one carbon double bond.
Multinutrient	A supplement containing a variety of essential or non-essential nutrients for either health or performance improvement.
n-3	Omega-3 fats. Fatty acids with a double bond at the third carbon atom from the methyl end of the carbon chain. Generally considered anti-inflammatory and including the essential fat alpha-linolenic acid (and it's DHA and EPA metabolites).

n-6	Omega-6 fats. Fatty acids with a double bond at the sixth carbon atom from the methyl end of the carbon chain. Generally considered pro-inflammatory and including the essential fat linoleic acid (and metabolites such as Arachidonic Acid [AA]).
Naturopathy	A complementary and alternative system of medicine encompassing drugless treatments such as nutrition, herbal medicine and supplementation.
Neuron	A nerve cell. Neurons transmit signals by electrical and chemical messengers.
Neurotransmitter	Chemicals that transmit a 'message' from a neuron (nerve cell) to another neuron, or a muscle cell or gland.
Norepinephrine	One of our major 'fight-or-flight' hormones. (Also known as *nor-adrenaline*).
NRV	Nutrient reference values. Australia and New Zealand government recommendations for nutrient intake.

Nutrient	Any of the various chemical compounds that 'nourish' the body.
Nutritional Ketosis	Sometimes abbreviated to NK. See 'Ketosis'.
Oestrogen	The sex hormone associated with female sexual characteristics. Also anti-inflammatory and associated with mood.
Oligosaccharide	A carbohydrate polymer consisting of 3-10 monosaccharides.
Oxaloacetate	An important intermediate for energy production (gluconeogenesis, urea cycle, glyoxylate cycle, amino acid synthesis, fatty acid synthesis and Krebs cycle).
Paleo Diet	A diet that seeks to emulate that if hunter-gatherer man. Typically includes vegetables, berries, fruit, tubers, meat, eggs, nuts and seeds and avoids grains, legumes, sugars and dairy.
Pathology	The study of disease or in the case of 'a pathology' a noun for the presence of disease or disorder.
Phospholipid	A lipid composed of two fatty acids and one phosphate group attached to a glycerol backbone. These form a major

[181]

	structural component of cell membranes.
PUFA	Polyunsaturated fatty acid. Contain more than one double bond.
Prebiotic	Non-digestible fibres and starches that feed beneficial bacteria in the gut.
Probiotic	Beneficial bacteria (and yeasts) found in supplements and fermented foods.
Progesterone	A steroid hormone that is primarily involved with the menstrual cycle, pregnancy and gestation and also is a neurotransmitter and important steroid hormone intermediate.
PSNS	Parasympathetic Nervous System. The 'rest-and-digest' system.
RBC	Red Blood Cell. Oxygen carrying cells lacking mitochondria (anaerobic only energy production).
RCT	Randomised Controlled Trial. A clinical trial in which people are randomised to receive either an intervention or control (usually a placebo). This reduces the risk of bias when allocating groups and controls for the placebo effect.

Rhinitis	Irritation and inflammation of the mucosa of the nose.
RS	Resistant Starch. Non-digestible long chain carbohydrates that feed beneficial bacteria in the gut.
Satiety	The feeling of satisfaction, fullness and sufficiency after eating.
Serotonin	Tryptophan derived, monoamine hormone associated with mood balance and smooth muscle function.
SFA	Saturated fatty acid. A fatty acid containing all single carbon bonds.
SNS	Sympathetic Nervous System. The 'fight-or-flight' system.
Staphylococcus	A genus of bacteria usually associated with infection, especially of the skin.
Steroid	A class of pro-hormones and hormones featuring four carbon rings. In the human body, this includes cholesterol, oestrogen, progesterone, testosterone, cortisol, aldosterone and other hormones.
Systematic Review	A study that collects and looks at multiple studies based on a defined search criteria and with exclusion and inclusion criteria based

	on the quality of evidence and applicability of terms.
Testosterone	A steroid hormone, known as the male sex hormone but found in both sexes. Associated with muscle growth and retention and some aspects of mood and libido.
Triglyceride/Triacylglycerol (TAG)	A lipid complex (a fat) made up of three fatty acids and a glycerol backbone.
Thermogenesis	The creation of heat in the body. A measure of metabolic activity.
Tocopherol	A class of methylated phenol chemicals making up part of the Vitamin E family including alpha, beta, delta and gamma forms.
Tocotrienol	A class of chemicals making up part of the Vitamin E family including alpha, beta, delta and gamma forms.
TUL/UL	Tolerable Upper Limit or Upper Limit. The highest level of daily nutrient intake that is likely to pose no risk of adverse health effects to almost all individuals in the general population. As intake increases above the UL, the risk of adverse effects increases.

Tumour	An abnormal growth of tissue that may be malignant (cancerous) or benign.
UC	Ulcerative Colitis. An autoimmune inflammatory bowel disease affecting the large bowel (colon).
USDA	The United States Department of Agriculture. Key roles include food safety and food nutrient analysis.
Vitamin	Essential organic compounds required in small amounts for survival and health.
VLCD	Very Low Calorie Diet.
VLCKD	Very Low Carbohydrate Ketogenic Diet.
'Warburg Effect'	The observation that most cancer cells predominantly produce energy through glycolysis (use of carbohydrate for fuel).
WHO	World Health Organisation. An agency of the United Nations concerned with public health.

APPENDICES

APPENDIX A: CHOLESTEROL

Cholesterol is a lipid molecule and modified sterol (steroid). It is an essential structural component of cell membranes required to maintain both membrane structural integrity and fluidity. Cholesterol is also the precursor for the steroid hormones, bile acids, and vitamin D.

Cholesterol relies on protein carriers produced by the liver. These are broadly categorised as low- and high-density lipoproteins (LDL and HDL respectively).

The 'Cholesterol Hypothesis' suggested that high levels of cholesterol were a cause of heart disease. This has since been disputed and roundly disproven and it is now more conventionally suggested that a ratio of HDL, LDL, TAG, total cholesterol and triglycerides (amongst other factors) are likely to be more indicative of an internal environment related to the development of cardiovascular disorders.

LDL transports cholesterol away from the liver to peripheral tissue and HDL brings it back to the liver for processing, conversion and excretion (via bile in the digestive tract). Thus, there needs to be an appropriate balance of HDL and LDL cholesterol, but neither are 'good' or 'bad'.

APPENDIX B: FOLATE VS FOLIC ACID

Summary

The synthetic form of folic acid used in many nutritional supplements can result in high levels of unmetabolised folic acid in the blood which may interfere with the actions of bio-active (natural) folate and may reduce immunity and increase the risk of cancer formation.

Key Points

- Folate and folic acid are often used interchangeably
- Commonly 'folate' refers to natural or bioactive forms of folate
- 'Folic acid' typically refers to synthetic folic acid (pteroylmonoglutamate)
- Synthetic folic acid is absorbed more quickly but metabolised more slowly leading to potentially damaging, high levels of folic acid in the blood.
- High levels of this unmetabolised folic acid are linked to reduction in ability to use folate and may impair immunity and be carcinogenic with long-term use

The form of folate that is used in food fortification and most dietary supplements is a synthetic form; *pteroylmonoglutamate*. In supplements and fortified foods, it is commonly called simply 'folic acid' and in common usage, the terms 'folate' and 'folic acid' are considered interchangeable. Folate in any form is not used directly within the body but is metabolised to a metabolically active co-enzyme, tetrahydrafolate (tetrahydrafolic acid).

dihydropteroate diphosphate + p-aminobenzoic acid (PABA)

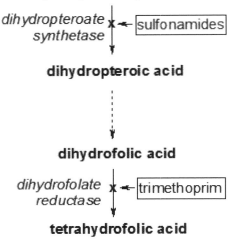

Pteroylmonoglutamate (synthetic folic acid) differs from the naturally occurring forms of folate in the diet because it is in an oxidized state and contains only one conjugated glutamate residue.

Interestingly it has much greater bioavailability than the natural folates and is rapidly absorbed from the intestine. This leads to high amounts of unmetabolised synthetic folic acid in the bloodstream.[209] Synthetic folates, when overloaded into the blood in this fashion, interfere with the metabolism, cellular transport, and regulatory functions of the natural folates that occur in the body by competing with them binding with enzymes, carrier proteins, and binding proteins.[210]

The folate receptor has a higher affinity for synthetic folic acid than for methyl-THF (the main natural form of folate that occurs in the blood.)

This may result in:

- Reduced levels of active folates for use as co-enzymes in brain function
- Down-regulation of folate receptors
- Change in gene expression of folate dependent enzymes

There is also considered to be a risk of liver capacity saturation with high dose folic acid supplementation, leading to higher levels of unmetabolised folic acid entering the general circulatory system. This would compound the potential negative effects mentioned above and may have direct effects on other functions such as immunity. [212, 213] Although high folate diets reduce the risk of cancer, high intakes of supplemental folic acid can increase carcinogenesis.[320] Many cancer drugs are anti-folates due to their ability to inhibit the growth of rapidly dividing cell types found in tumours.

IS NATURAL FOLATE SUPPLEMENTATION JUSTIFIED?

The benefits of folate supplementation in reducing neural tube defects in babies is undeniable, and the vital role of folate for overall health is clear, but the potential risks associated with synthetic folic acid make natural folates a more prudent supplemental choice.

Natural folate supplements using L-5-methyl-THF may also reduce the effects of Vitamin B12 deficiency masking (folic acid taken in large doses can mask the effects of a B12 deficiency so that it often remains undiagnosed for a longer time, resulting in neural damage) and may reduce interactions with drugs that inhibit dihydrofolate reductase.[321]

Recent research has shown that the actual amount of folate in foods is approximately 25% lower than what was previously thought.[322]

CONCLUSION

Supplementing with synthetic folic acid forms may put some people at risk. People not eating the recommended 6+ servings of vegetables per day, pregnant and breastfeeding women, and active or highly stressed individuals, should use a bio-active (methylated) form of folate such as L5-MTHF.

APPENDIX C: SELECTED WHOLE FOOD SUPPLEMENT INGREDIENTS

ACEROLA

The fruit of the acerola tree has approximately 10-50 times more Vitamin C by weight than oranges along with other antioxidant bioflavonoids and magnesium, pantothenic acid and Vitamin A.

ALPHA-LIPOIC ACID

Alpha lipoic acid is a type of fatty acid. It's found in every cell and helps to generate energy and aids the conversion of glucose to energy. Alpha lipoic acid also functions as an antioxidant and unlike most antioxidants works in both water and fatty tissues so has a broad spectrum of antioxidant actions.

APPLE POWDER:

Apples are a highly nutritious food and provide fibre (in the form of pectin) that feeds the good bacteria that help support optimal digestive health.

BARLEY LEAF

Barley leaf is a highly nutritious food. It contains a range of vitamins, minerals and amino acids and is considered a great supportive food for general health.

BEETROOT

Beets are a high antioxidant food, also very high in dietary nitrates. Dietary nitrates have been demonstrated to help combat fatigue and improve physical performance.

BETA GLUCANS

Beta glucans are a type of soluble fibre from many plants. They are now allowed a 'heart healthy' label in many jurisdictions for their purported effects on improving cholesterol profiles. Beta glucans are also considered to improve immune function.

BILBERRY

Bilberry is another high antioxidant berry (closely related to the blueberry and cranberry). It has a long traditional use, especially for improving vision. It is high in anthocyanosides that may benefit the retina of the eye and aid connective tissue formation and reduce inflammation.

BIOFLAVONOIDS

Bioflavonoids are additional health promoting compounds found in abundance in citrus fruits. They are thought to aid the actions of Vitamin C and other antioxidants. Bioflavonoids may improve vein and capillary strength and reduce bruising.[323]

BLACKCURRANT EXTRACT

New Zealand blackcurrants are considered one of the highest antioxidants berries.

BROCCOLI SPROUTS

Broccoli is a highly nutritious vegetable and the sprouts of the broccoli seed have the added benefit of containing glucoraphanin. Glucoraphanin is converted to an active compound sulfurophane which aids natural detox pathways and act as a powerful antioxidant in the body.

CACAO

Theobroma cocoa – the cocoa or cacao plant is known as the 'food of the gods'. Cacao is one of the foods richest in health promoting antioxidants that may help to reduce damage to cells and that might reduce UV related damage.[324] Look for a high quality raw cacao.

CAMU CAMU

Camu camu is another highly nutritious berry from the Amazon that has an extraordinarily high Vitamin C content along with natural bioflavonoids that aid the antioxidant actions of Vitamin C.

CARROT ROOT

Carrots are foods naturally high in antioxidant carotenoids that help to improve night vision and support eye health. Carrots also provide fibre that supports gut health.

DANDELION

Dandelion is a traditional culinary vegetable and herb that is extraordinarily nutritious. It is high in vitamins A, C, D and B complex as well as iron, magnesium, zinc, potassium, manganese, copper, choline, calcium, boron and silicon. Traditionally it has been used to support the health of the liver, kidneys and the general digestive system.

GINGER

Ginger is a highly nutritive herb with a long history of traditional medical and culinary use.

GOJI

The berry of the Lycium chinensis plant, also known as Wolfberry has a long history of traditional use, especially in traditional Chinese medicine (TCM). It is considered in TCM to be nourishing for the kidneys, liver and lungs. It has been used traditionally to treat dry skin, dizziness, poor libido, low back pain and a dry cough. It is a highly nutritious berry, very high in antioxidants.

GRAPESEED EXTRACT

Grape seeds provide high levels of 'pro-anthocyanins' that aid the antioxidant capacity of the body and are believed to have activity against both fat soluble and water soluble free-radicals.

There is good evidence that these compounds reduce leg pain and swelling related to chronic venous insufficiency, PMS and reduce swelling associated with injury and surgery.[325, 326]

Kelp

Kelp is a type of seaweed that is a nutritious food and that forms a regular part of the diet in many parts of the world including Japan, Alaska and Hawaii. It is a good source of folate, and iodine. Iodine is important to enable the body to produce thyroid hormones that regulate metabolic rate.

Pea Protein

Protein is the building block for all cells, tissue and organs in the body and so is essential for growing bodies to develop to their best potential. Protein may also aid stability of energy levels, and help to encourage healthy eating patterns. Look for a high quality Pea Protein Isolate.

Pineapple & Papaya juice extracts

Papaya, like most fruits, are highly nutritive foods for general health. Two enzymes, in particular, are found in papaya and pineapple; bromelain and papain. These enzymes can be absorbed into the body[327] and help reduce inflammation and pain.[328]

Probiotics

Probiotics like acidophilus and bifidobacteria are beneficial bacteria that help to protect the gut from harmful bacteria and yeasts. Probiotics are useful to help the population of the gut with helpful bacteria, while crowding out the harmful. Antibiotics disturb the balance of bacteria and probiotics help to redress this imbalance. Probiotic supplements reduce severity and duration of antibiotic related, infectious, and persistent diarrhoea in children[329-332] and help to prevent upper respiratory tract infections.[333]

PSYLLIUM HUSK

Psyllium is a soluble fibre from the plant *Plantago ovata.* Soluble fibres help to support the healthy bacterial balance in the gut, which helps to support immune and overall health. Systematic reviews of the evidence suggest that psyllium fibre is also effective for aiding regularity and bowel health and reducing constipation.[334-336]

RED MARINE ALGAE

Red marine algae are a source of highly bioavailable, all-natural calcium to support the growth and development of bones and support nervous system health.

SPINACH

Spinach is a nutritive vegetable that is high in vitamins A, C, E and K and folate and B vitamins along with magnesium, manganese, calcium, potassium and dietary fibre.

SPIRULINA AND CHLORELLA

Spirulina are members of a blue-green algae family that grows in the wild in Mexico and in Africa. It is a highly nutritious food has been traditionally used by indigenous people in Mexico and Central Africa. Spirulina contains high levels of B vitamins, beta-carotene, other carotenoids, gamma-linoleic acid, and minerals such as calcium, iron, magnesium, zinc, manganese and potassium. Spirulina is typically used for general nutritional support and may have additional benefits. Chlorella helps to reduce blood pressure, lower cholesterol, accelerate wound healing, reduce symptoms of fibromyalgia and enhance immune function.[337]

Highly preliminary evidence suggests Spirulina may help to reduce the certain types of cancers[338] and reduce symptoms of allergy.[339, 340]

SUNFLOWER LECITHIN

Lecithin contains phosphatidylcholine (PC) a substance that forms part of the cell membrane. It also provides choline, a precursor of acetylcholine, a major neurotransmitter (a chemical 'signal' between cells). PC supports the healthy development of all cells, especially cells of the brain and central nervous system and aid the production of acetylcholine.

Soy lecithin is the most common form available. However, sunflower lecithin is also relatively common and is useful for those suffering from a soy intolerance or allergy.

WHEATGRASS

Wheatgrass is a highly nutritious food. It contains a range of vitamins, minerals and amino acids and is considered a great supportive food for general health. It is important to note that wheat grass does not contain gluten, as the gluten is contained only in the wheat grain and not the growing shoots of the wheat grass.

APPENDIX D: CALORIE CALCULATION

The Harris–Benedict equations as revised by Roza and Shizgal.[341]

Men	BMR = 88.362 + (13.397 x weight in kg) + (4.799 x height in cm) - (5.677 x age in years)
Women	BMR = 447.593 + (9.247 x weight in kg) + (3.098 x height in cm) - (4.330 x age in years)

The 95% confidence range for men is ±210.5 kcal/day, and ±201.0 kcal/day for women.

References

1. Flegal, K.M., et al., *Prevalence of obesity and trends in the distribution of body mass index among US adults, 1999-2010.* JAMA, 2012. **307**(5): p. 491-497.
2. New Zealand Ministry of Health. *Obesity Data and Statistics.* 2013; Available from: http://www.health.govt.nz/nz-health-statistics/health-statistics-and-data-sets/obesity-data-and-stats.
3. Whiting, D.R., et al., *IDF Diabetes Atlas: Global estimates of the prevalence of diabetes for 2011 and 2030.* Diabetes Research and Clinical Practice, 2011. **94**(3): p. 311-321.
4. Peeters, A., et al., *Obesity in Adulthood and Its Consequences for Life Expectancy: A Life-Table Analysis.* Annals of Internal Medicine, 2003. **138**(1): p. 24-32.
5. Olshansky, S.J., et al., *A Potential Decline in Life Expectancy in the United States in the 21st Century.* New England Journal of Medicine, 2005. **352**(11): p. 1138-1145.
6. Stewart, S.T., D.M. Cutler, and A.B. Rosen, *Forecasting the Effects of Obesity and Smoking on U.S. Life Expectancy.* New England Journal of Medicine, 2009. **361**(23): p. 2252-2260.
7. Centers for Disease Control and Prevention, *Trends in intake of energy and macronutrients--United States, 1971-2000.* MMWR. Morbidity and mortality weekly report, 2004. **53**(4): p. 80.
8. Diabetes New Zealand. *Essentials of Healthy Eating - The Main Food Groups.* 2014 3/3/2015]; Available from: http://www.diabetes.org.nz/food_and_nutrition/the_essentials/main_food_groups.
9. Gillespie, S.J., K.D. Kulkarni, and A.E. Daly, *Using Carbohydrate Counting in Diabetes Clinical Practice.* Journal of the American Dietetic Association. **98**(8): p. 897-905.
10. Kulkarni, K.D., *Carbohydrate Counting: A Practical Meal-Planning Option for People With Diabetes.* Clinical Diabetes, 2005. **23**(3): p. 120-122.
11. Dietitians Association of Australia. *Nutrient Reference Values.* 2013 10/3/2015]; Available from: http://daa.asn.au/for-the-public/smart-eating-for-you/nutrition-a-z/nutrient-reference-values-nrvs/.

12. Roberts, D., *Carbohydrates and Dietary Fibre*. 1999, National Heart Foundation.

13. Gerstein, H.C., *Dysglycaemia: a cardiovascular risk factor.* Diabetes Research and Clinical Practice, 1998. **40, Supplement 1**: p. S9-S14.

14. Sarwar, N., et al., *Markers of dysglycaemia and risk of coronary heart disease in people without diabetes: Reykjavik prospective study and systematic review.* PLoS Med, 2010. **7**(5): p. e1000278.

15. Anand, S., et al., *Glucose levels are associated with cardiovascular disease and death in an international cohort of normal glycaemic and dysglycaemic men and women: the EpiDREAM cohort study.* European Journal of Preventive Cardiology, 2012. **19**(4): p. 755-764.

16. Liu, S., et al., *A prospective study of dietary glycemic load, carbohydrate intake, and risk of coronary heart disease in US women.* The American Journal of Clinical Nutrition, 2000. **71**(6): p. 1455-1461.

17. World Health Organisation, *Carbohydrates in Human Nutrition*. 1998, World Health Organisation or the Food and Agriculture Organisation of the United Nations.

18. Mann, J., et al., *FAO//WHO Scientific Update on carbohydrates in human nutrition: conclusions.* Eur J Clin Nutr, 2007. **61**(S1): p. S132-S137.

19. Wheeler, M.L., et al., *Macronutrients, Food Groups, and Eating Patterns in the Management of Diabetes A systematic review of the literature, 2010.* Diabetes Care, 2012. **35**(2): p. 434-445.

20. Westman, E.C., *Is dietary carbohydrate essential for human nutrition?* The American Journal of Clinical Nutrition, 2002. **75**(5): p. 951-953.

21. Paoli, A., et al., *Beyond weight loss: a review of the therapeutic uses of very-low-carbohydrate (ketogenic) diets.* European journal of clinical nutrition, 2013. **67**(8): p. 789-796.

22. Sumithran, P. and J. Proietto, *Ketogenic diets for weight loss: A review of their principles, safety and efficacy.* Obesity Research & Clinical Practice, 2008. **2**(1): p. 1-13.

23.   Feinman, R.D. and E.J. Fine, *"A calorie is a calorie" violates the second law of thermodynamics.* Nutrition Journal, 2004. **3**: p. 9-9.

24.   Buchholz, A.C. and D.A. Schoeller, *Is a calorie a calorie?* The American Journal of Clinical Nutrition, 2004. **79**(5): p. 899S-906S.

25.   Holmberg, S., A. Thelin, and E.-L. Stiernström, *Food Choices and Coronary Heart Disease: A Population Based Cohort Study of Rural Swedish Men with 12 Years of Follow-up.* International Journal of Environmental Research and Public Health, 2009. **6**(10): p. 2626-2638.

26.   Larsson, S.C., et al., *Calcium and dairy food intakes are inversely associated with colorectal cancer risk in the Cohort of Swedish Men.* The American Journal of Clinical Nutrition, 2006. **83**(3): p. 667-673.

27.   Berkey, C.S., et al., *Milk, dairy fat, dietary calcium, and weight gain: A longitudinal study of adolescents.* Archives of Pediatrics & Adolescent Medicine, 2005. **159**(6): p. 543-550.

28.   Kratz, M., T. Baars, and S. Guyenet, *The relationship between high-fat dairy consumption and obesity, cardiovascular, and metabolic disease.* Eur J Nutr, 2013. **52**(1): p. 1-24.

29.   Hooper, L., et al., *Reduced or modified dietary fat for preventing cardiovascular disease.* Cochrane Database Syst Rev, 2011(7): p. CD002137.

30.   Siri-Tarino, P.W., et al., *Meta-analysis of prospective cohort studies evaluating the association of saturated fat with cardiovascular disease.* The American journal of clinical nutrition, 2010. **91**(3): p. 535-546.

31.   Mente, A., et al., *A systematic review of the evidence supporting a causal link between dietary factors and coronary heart disease.* Arch Intern Med, 2009. **169**(7): p. 659-69.

32.   Mozaffarian, D., R. Micha, and S. Wallace, *Effects on coronary heart disease of increasing polyunsaturated fat in place of saturated fat: a systematic review and meta-analysis of randomized controlled trials.* PLoS Med, 2010. **7**(3): p. e1000252.

33.   Jakobsen, M.U., et al., *Major types of dietary fat and risk of coronary heart disease: a pooled analysis of 11 cohort studies.* Am J Clin Nutr, 2009. **89**(5): p. 1425-32.

34.   Skeaff, C.M. and J. Miller, *Dietary fat and coronary heart disease: summary of evidence from prospective cohort and randomised controlled trials.* Annals of Nutrition & Metabolism, 2009. **55**(1-3): p. 173-201.

35.   Turpeinen, O., et al., *Dietary prevention of coronary heart disease: the Finnish Mental Hospital Study.* International Journal of Epidemiology, 1979. **8**(2): p. 99-118.

36.   Ramsden, C.E., et al., *Use of dietary linoleic acid for secondary prevention of coronary heart disease and death: evaluation of recovered data from the Sydney Diet Heart Study and updated meta-analysis.* BMJ, 2013. **346**.

37.   Madsen, L. and K. Kristiansen, *Of mice and men.* 2012.

38.   Institute of Medicine of the National Academies, *Dietary reference intakes for water, potassium, sodium, chloride and sulphate.* 2005: Washington, D.C.

39.   Graudal, N., T. Hubeck-Graudal, and G. Jurgens, *Effects of low sodium diet versus high sodium diet on blood pressure, renin, aldosterone, catecholamines, cholesterol, and triglyceride.* Cochrane Database Syst Rev, 2011. **11**.

40.   Taylor, R.S., et al., *Reduced Dietary Salt for the Prevention of Cardiovascular Disease: A Meta-Analysis of Randomized Controlled Trials (Cochrane Review).* American Journal of Hypertension, 2011. **24**(8): p. 843-853.

41.   Institute of Medicine of the National Academies, *Sodium intake in populations: Assessment of evidence.* 2013: Washington, D.C.

42.   Institute of Medicine, *Sodium Intake in Populations: Assessment of Evidence.* 2013, National Academies Press: Washington DC. USA.

43.   Graudal, N., et al., *Compared With Usual Sodium Intake, Low- and Excessive-Sodium Diets Are Associated With Increased Mortality: A Meta-Analysis.* American Journal of Hypertension, 2014.

44.   Alderman, M.H. and H.W. Cohen, *Dietary Sodium Intake and Cardiovascular Mortality: Controversy Resolved?* American Journal of Hypertension, 2012. **25**(7): p. 727-34.

45.   McLean, R., et al., *1051 Estimates of New Zealand Population Sodium Intake: Use of Spot Urine in the 2008/09 Adult*

Nutrition Survey. Journal of Hypertension, 2012. **30**: p. e306 10.1097/01.hjh.0000420510.93854.ca.

46.   Thomson, B.M., R.W. Vannoort, and R.M. Haslemore, *Dietary exposure and trends of exposure to nutrient elements iodine, iron, selenium and sodium from the 2003–4 New Zealand Total Diet Survey.* British Journal of Nutrition, 2008. **99**(03): p. 614-625.

47.   Thomson, C.D., *Selenium and iodine intakes and status in New Zealand and Australia.* British Journal of Nutrition, 2004. **91**(05): p. 661-672.

48.   Mummert, A., et al., *Stature and robusticity during the agricultural transition: evidence from the bioarchaeological record.* Econ Hum Biol, 2011. **9**(3): p. 284-301.

49.   Sinclair, H.M., *The Diet of Canadian Indians and Eskimos.* Proceedings of the Nutrition Society, 1953. **12**(01): p. 69-82.

50.   O'Dea, K., *Westernisation, insulin resistance and diabetes in Australian aborigines.* The Medical journal of Australia, 1991. **155**(4): p. 258-264.

51.   Speth, J.D. and K.A. Spielmann, *Energy source, protein metabolism, and hunter-gatherer subsistence strategies.* Journal of Anthropological Archaeology, 1983. **2**(1): p. 1-31.

52.   Domínguez-Rodrigo, M., *Hunting and scavenging by early humans: the state of the debate.* Journal of World Prehistory, 2002. **16**(1): p. 1-54.

53.   Ströhle, A. and A. Hahn, *Diets of modern hunter-gatherers vary substantially in their carbohydrate content depending on ecoenvironments: results from an ethnographic analysis.* Nutrition Research. **31**(6): p. 429-435.

54.   Braakhuis, A., et al., *Physiological analysis of the metabolic typing diet in professional rugby union players.* NZ Journal of Sports Medicine, 2007.

55.   Falchi, M., et al., *Low copy number of the salivary amylase gene predisposes to obesity.* Nat Genet, 2014. **46**(5): p. 492-7.

56.   Perry, G.H., et al., *Diet and the evolution of human amylase gene copy number variation.* Nature genetics, 2007. **39**(10): p. 1256-1260.

57.   Mandel, A.L. and P.A.S. Breslin, *High Endogenous Salivary Amylase Activity Is Associated with Improved Glycemic*

[204]

Homeostasis following Starch Ingestion in Adults. The Journal of Nutrition, 2012. **142**(5): p. 853-858.

58.   Nakamura, Y., et al., *Low-carbohydrate diets and cardiovascular and total mortality in Japanese: a 29-year follow-up of NIPPON DATA80.* Br J Nutr, 2014. **112**(6): p. 916-24.

59.   Davis, D.R., M.D. Epp, and H.D. Riordan, *Changes in USDA Food Composition Data for 43 Garden Crops, 1950 to 1999.* Journal of the American College of Nutrition, 2004. **23**(6): p. 669-682.

60.   University of Otago and Ministry of Health., *A Focus on Nutrition: Key findings of the 2008/09 New Zealand Adult Nutrition Survey.* 2011: Wellington.

61.   Hellstrom, P.M., *Satiety signals and obesity.* Curr Opin Gastroenterol, 2013. **29**(2): p. 222-7.

62.   Naslund, E. and P.M. Hellstrom, *Appetite signaling: from gut peptides and enteric nerves to brain.* Physiol Behav, 2007. **92**(1-2): p. 256-62.

63.   Maljaars, J., *Overeating makes the gut grow fonder; new insights in gastrointestinal satiety signaling in obesity.* Curr Opin Gastroenterol, 2013. **29**(2): p. 177-83.

64.   Layman, D.K. and J.I. Baum, *Dietary Protein Impact on Glycemic Control during Weight Loss.* The Journal of Nutrition, 2004. **134**(4): p. 968S-973S.

65.   Layman, D.K., et al., *A Reduced Ratio of Dietary Carbohydrate to Protein Improves Body Composition and Blood Lipid Profiles during Weight Loss in Adult Women.* The Journal of Nutrition, 2003. **133**(2): p. 411-417.

66.   Piatti, P.M., et al., *Hypocaloric high-protein diet improves glucose oxidation and spares lean body mass: Comparison to hypocaloric high-carbohydrate diet.* Metabolism, 1994. **43**(12): p. 1481-1487.

67.   Farnsworth, E., et al., *Effect of a high-protein, energy-restricted diet on body composition, glycemic control, and lipid concentrations in overweight and obese hyperinsulinemic men and women.* The American Journal of Clinical Nutrition, 2003. **78**(1): p. 31-39.

68.   Noakes, M., et al., *Effect of an energy-restricted, high-protein, low-fat diet relative to a conventional high-carbohydrate, low-*

[205]

fat diet on weight loss, body composition, nutritional status, and markers of cardiovascular health in obese women. The American Journal of Clinical Nutrition, 2005. **81**(6): p. 1298-1306.

69. Labayen, I., et al. *Effects of protein vs. carbohydrate-rich diets on fuel utilisation in obese women during weight loss*. in *Forum of Nutrition*. 2002.

70. Keller, U., *Dietary proteins in obesity and in diabetes.* International Journal for Vitamin and Nutrition Research, 2011. **81**(23): p. 125-133.

71. Veldhorst, M.A., M.S. Westerterp-Plantenga, and K.R. Westerterp, *Gluconeogenesis and energy expenditure after a high-protein, carbohydrate-free diet.* The American Journal of Clinical Nutrition, 2009. **90**(3): p. 519-526.

72. Westerterp, K.R., *Diet induced thermogenesis.* Nutrition & Metabolism, 2004. **1**(1): p. 5.

73. Johnston, C.S., C.S. Day, and P.D. Swan, *Postprandial Thermogenesis Is Increased 100% on a High-Protein, Low-Fat Diet versus a High-Carbohydrate, Low-Fat Diet in Healthy, Young Women.* Journal of the American College of Nutrition, 2002. **21**(1): p. 55-61.

74. Robinson, S.M., et al., *Protein turnover and thermogenesis in response to high-protein and high-carbohydrate feeding in men.* The American Journal of Clinical Nutrition, 1990. **52**(1): p. 72-80.

75. Roberts, S.B. and V.R. Young, *Energy costs of fat and protein deposition in the human infant.* The American Journal of Clinical Nutrition, 1988. **48**(4): p. 951-5.

76. Luscombe, N., et al., *Effects of energy-restricted diets containing increased protein on weight loss, resting energy expenditure, and the thermic effect of feeding in type 2 diabetes.* Diabetes Care, 2002. **25**(4): p. 652-657.

77. Halton, T.L. and F.B. Hu, *The Effects of High Protein Diets on Thermogenesis, Satiety and Weight Loss: A Critical Review.* Journal of the American College of Nutrition, 2004. **23**(5): p. 373-385.

78. Johnstone, A.M., et al., *Effects of a high-protein ketogenic diet on hunger, appetite, and weight loss in obese men feeding ad*

libitum. The American Journal of Clinical Nutrition, 2008. **87**(1): p. 44-55.

79.   Tendler, D., et al., *The Effect of a Low-Carbohydrate, Ketogenic Diet on Nonalcoholic Fatty Liver Disease: A Pilot Study.* Digestive Diseases and Sciences, 2007. **52**(2): p. 589-93.

80.   Nielsen, J.V., et al., *Low carbohydrate diet in type 1 diabetes, long-term improvement and adherence: A clinical audit.* Diabetology & metabolic syndrome, 2012. **4**(1): p. 23.

81.   Yancy, W., et al., *A low-carbohydrate, ketogenic diet to treat type 2 diabetes.* Nutrition & Metabolism, 2005. **2**(1): p. 34.

82.   Fine, E.J., et al., *Targeting insulin inhibition as a metabolic therapy in advanced cancer: A pilot safety and feasibility dietary trial in 10 patients.* Nutrition, 2012.

83.   Krikorian, R., et al., *Dietary ketosis enhances memory in mild cognitive impairment.* Neurobiology of Aging, 2012. **33**(2): p. 425.e19-425.e27.

84.   Shai, I., et al., *Weight loss with a low-carbohydrate, mediterranean, or low-fat diet.* New England Journal of Medicine, 2008. **359**(3): p. 229-241.

85.   Ebbeling, C.B., et al., *Effects of dietary composition on energy expenditure during weight-loss maintenance.* JAMA, 2012. **307**(24): p. 2627-2634.

86.   McAuley, K.A., et al., *Long-term effects of popular dietary approaches on weight loss and features of insulin resistance.* International Journal of Obesity, 2006. **30**(2): p. 342-349.

87.   Sikaris, K., *Cholesterol vs fat vs glucose*, in *The why and how of low carb eating.* 2014: Auckland.

88.   Westman, E.C., et al., *Effect of a low-carbohydrate, ketogenic diet program compared to a low-fat diet on fasting lipoprotein subclasses.* International Journal of Cardiology, 2006. **110**(2): p. 212-216.

89.   Benoit, F.L., R.L. Martin, and R.H. Watten, *Changes in body composition during weight reduction in obesity. Balance studies comparing effects of fasting and a ketogenic diet.* Annals Of Internal Medicine, 1965. **63**(4): p. 604-612.

90.   Dreyer, H.C., et al., *Leucine-enriched essential amino acid and carbohydrate ingestion following resistance exercise enhances mTOR signaling and protein synthesis in human muscle.* Vol. 294. 2008. E392-E400.

91.	Tipton, K.D., et al., *Postexercise net protein synthesis in human muscle from orally administered amino acids.* Am J Physiol, 1999. **276**(4): p. E628-E634.

92.	Anthony, J.C., et al., *Signaling Pathways Involved in Translational Control of Protein Synthesis in Skeletal Muscle by Leucine.* The Journal of Nutrition, 2001. **131**(3): p. 856S-860S.

93.	Norton, L.E. and D.K. Layman, *Leucine Regulates Translation Initiation of Protein Synthesis in Skeletal Muscle after Exercise.* The Journal of Nutrition, 2006. **136**(2): p. 533S-537S.

94.	Koopman, R., et al., *Combined ingestion of protein and free leucine with carbohydrate increases postexercise muscle protein synthesis in vivo in male subjects.* Am J Physiol Endocrinol Metab, 2005. **288**(4): p. E645-E653.

95.	Luscombe-Marsh, N.D., et al., *Carbohydrate-restricted diets high in either monounsaturated fat or protein are equally effective at promoting fat loss and improving blood lipids.* The American Journal of Clinical Nutrition, 2005. **81**(4): p. 762-772.

96.	Ullrich, I.H., P.J. Peters, and M. Albrink, *Effect of low-carbohydrate diets high in either fat or protein on thyroid function, plasma insulin, glucose, and triglycerides in healthy young adults.* Journal of the American College of Nutrition, 1985. **4**(4): p. 451-459.

97.	Bligh, H.F., et al., *Plant-rich mixed meals based on Palaeolithic diet principles have a dramatic impact on incretin, peptide YY and satiety response, but show little effect on glucose and insulin homeostasis: an acute-effects randomised study.* Br J Nutr, 2015. **113**: p. 574-84.

98.	Jönsson, T., et al., *Subjective satiety and other experiences of a Paleolithic diet compared to a diabetes diet in patients with type 2 diabetes.* Nutrition Journal, 2013. **12**: p. 105.

99.	Jonsson, T., et al., *A paleolithic diet is more satiating per calorie than a mediterranean-like diet in individuals with ischemic heart disease.* Nutr Metab (Lond), 2010. **7**: p. 85.

100.	Masharani, U., et al., *Metabolic and physiologic effects from consuming a hunter-gatherer (Paleolithic)-type diet in type 2 diabetes.* Eur J Clin Nutr, 2015.

101.	Frassetto, L.A., et al., *Metabolic and physiologic improvements from consuming a paleolithic, hunter-gatherer type diet.* Eur J Clin Nutr, 2009. **63**(8): p. 947-955.

[208]

102. Mellberg, C., et al., *Long-term effects of a Palaeolithic-type diet in obese postmenopausal women: a 2-year randomized trial.* Eur J Clin Nutr, 2014. **68**(3): p. 350-357.

103. Ryberg, M., et al., *A Palaeolithic-type diet causes strong tissue-specific effects on ectopic fat deposition in obese postmenopausal women.* Journal of Internal Medicine, 2013. **274**(1): p. 67-76.

104. Eaton, S.B., M. Konner, and M. Shostak, *Stone agers in the fast lane: Chronic degenerative diseases in evolutionary perspective.* The American Journal of Medicine, 1988. **84**(4): p. 739-749.

105. O'Keefe, J.J.H., et al., *Optimal low-density lipoprotein is 50 to 70 mg/dlLower is better and physiologically normal.* Journal of the American College of Cardiology, 2004. **43**(11): p. 2142-2146.

106. O'Dea, K., *Westernization and non-insulin-dependent diabetes in Australian Aborigines.* Ethnicity & disease, 1991. **1**(2): p. 171-187.

107. Horne, B.D., J.B. Muhlestein, and J.L. Anderson, *Health effects of intermittent fasting: hormesis or harm? A systematic review.* American Journal of Clinical Nutrition, 2015. **102**(2): p. 464-470.

108. Rothschild, J., et al., *Time-restricted feeding and risk of metabolic disease: a review of human and animal studies.* Nutrition Reviews, 2014. **72**(5): p. 308-318.

109. Chaouachi, A., et al., *The effects of Ramadan intermittent fasting on athletic performance: Recommendations for the maintenance of physical fitness.* Journal of Sports Sciences, 2012. **30**(Supp 1): p. S53-S73.

110. Shephard, R.J., *Ramadan and Sport: Minimizing Effects Upon the Observant Athlete.* Sports Medicine, 2013. **43**(12): p. 1217-1241 25p.

111. Ilomaki, J., et al., *Alcohol Consumption, Dementia and Cognitive Decline: An Overview of Systematic Reviews.* Current Clinical Pharmacology, 2015. **10**(3): p. 204-212.

112. Knott, C., S. Bell, and A. Britton, *Alcohol Consumption and the Risk of Type 2 Diabetes: A Systematic Review and Dose-Response Meta-analysis of More Than 1.9 Million Individuals*

From 38 Observational Studies. Diabetes Care, 2015. **38**(9): p. 1804-1812.

113.   Howard, A.A., J.H. Arnsten, and M.N. Gourevitch, *Effect of alcohol consumption on diabetes mellitus: a systematic review.* Annals of Internal Medicine, 2004. **140**(3): p. 211.

114.   Schrieks, I.C., et al., *The effect of alcohol consumption on insulin sensitivity and glycemic status: a systematic review and meta-analysis of intervention studies.* Diabetes Care, 2015. **38**(4): p. 723-732.

115.   Roerecke, M. and J. Rehm, *The cardioprotective association of average alcohol consumption and ischaemic heart disease: a systematic review and meta-analysis.* Addiction, 2012. **107**(7): p. 1246-1260.

116.   Roerecke, M. and J. Rehm, *Alcohol consumption, drinking patterns, and ischemic heart disease: a narrative review of meta-analyses and a systematic review and meta-analysis of the impact of heavy drinking occasions on risk for moderate drinkers.* BMC Medicine, 2014. **12**: p. 182-182.

117.   Ronksley, P.E., et al., *Association of alcohol consumption with selected cardiovascular disease outcomes: a systematic review and meta-analysis.* BMJ (Clinical Research Ed.), 2011. **342**: p. d671-d671.

118.   Brien, S.E., et al., *Effect of alcohol consumption on biological markers associated with risk of coronary heart disease: systematic review and meta-analysis of interventional studies.* BMJ (Clinical Research Ed.), 2011. **342**: p. d636-d636.

119.   Chen, L., et al., *Alcohol consumption and the risk of nasopharyngeal carcinoma: a systematic review.* Nutrition & Cancer, 2009. **61**(1): p. 1-15.

120.   Jayasekara, H., et al., *Alcohol Consumption Over Time and Risk of Death: A Systematic Review and Meta-Analysis.* American Journal of Epidemiology, 2014. **179**(9): p. 1049-1059.

121.   Buja, A., et al., *Is moderate alcohol consumption a risk factor for kidney function decline? A systematic review of observational studies.* Journal of Renal Nutrition, 2014. **24**(4): p. 224-235.

122.   Sayon-Orea, C., M.A. Martinez-Gonzalez, and M. Bes-Rastrollo, *Alcohol consumption and body weight: a systematic review.* Nutrition Reviews, 2011. **69**(8): p. 419-431.

[210]

123.   Mazzaglia, G., et al., *Exploring the relationship between alcohol consumption and non-fatal or fatal stroke: a systematic review.* Addiction, 2001. **96**(12): p. 1743-1756.

124.   Patra, J., et al., *Alcohol consumption and the risk of morbidity and mortality for different stroke types--a systematic review and meta-analysis.* BMC Public Health, 2010. **10**: p. 258-258.

125.   de Menezes, R.F., A. Bergmann, and L.C.S. Thuler, *Alcohol consumption and risk of cancer: a systematic literature review.* Asian Pacific Journal Of Cancer Prevention: APJCP, 2013. **14**(9): p. 4965-4972.

126.   Huang, Y.-H., et al., *Association between alcohol consumption and the risk of ovarian cancer: a meta-analysis of prospective observational studies.* BMC Public Health, 2015. **15**(1): p. 1-12.

127.   Zhen-Yu, Q., et al., *Alcohol Consumption and Risk of Glioma: A Meta-Analysis of 19 Observational Studies.* Nutrients, 2014. **6**(2): p. 504-516.

128.   Zhu, J.Z., et al., *Systematic review with meta-analysis: alcohol consumption and the risk of colorectal adenoma.* Alimentary Pharmacology & Therapeutics, 2014. **40**(4): p. 325-337.

129.   Taylor, B., J. Rehm, and G. Gmel, *Moderate alcohol consumption and the gastrointestinal tract.* Digestive Diseases (Basel, Switzerland), 2005. **23**(3-4): p. 170-176.

130.   White, I.R., *The level of alcohol consumption at which all-cause mortality is least.* Journal Of Clinical Epidemiology, 1999. **52**(10): p. 967-975.

131.   van Dam, R.M. and F.B. Hu, *Coffee consumption and risk of type 2 diabetes: A systematic review.* JAMA, 2005. **294**(1): p. 97-104.

132.   Muley, A., P. Muley, and M. Shah, *Coffee to Reduce Risk of Type 2 Diabetes? : A Systematic Review.* Current Diabetes Reviews, 2012. **8**(3): p. 162-168.

133.   Ding, M., et al., *Caffeinated and Decaffeinated Coffee Consumption and Risk of Type 2 Diabetes: A Systematic Review and a Dose-Response Meta-analysis.* Diabetes Care, 2014. **37**(2): p. 569-586.

134.   Huxley, R., et al., *Coffee, decaffeinated coffee, and tea consumption in relation to incident type 2 diabetes mellitus: A systematic review with meta-analysis.* Archives of Internal Medicine, 2009. **169**(22): p. 2053-2063.

135.   Mesas, A.E., et al., *The effect of coffee on blood pressure and cardiovascular disease in hypertensive individuals: a systematic review and meta-analysis.* The American Journal of Clinical Nutrition, 2011.

136.   Steffen, M., et al., *The effect of coffee consumption on blood pressure and the development of hypertension: a systematic review and meta-analysis.* Journal of Hypertension, 2012. **30**(12): p. 2245-2254.

137.   Zhang, Z., et al., *Habitual coffee consumption and risk of hypertension: a systematic review and meta-analysis of prospective observational studies.* The American Journal of Clinical Nutrition, 2011. **93**(6): p. 1212-1219.

138.   Ding, M., et al., *Long-Term Coffee Consumption and Risk of Cardiovascular Disease: A Systematic Review and a Dose-Response Meta-Analysis of Prospective Cohort Studies.* Circulation, 2013.

139.   Saab, S., et al., *Impact of coffee on liver diseases: a systematic review.* Liver International, 2014. **34**(4): p. 495-504.

140.   Zhang, Y.P., et al., *Systematic review with meta-analysis: coffee consumption and the risk of gallstone disease.* Alimentary Pharmacology & Therapeutics, 2015. **42**(6): p. 637-648.

141.   Lee, D.R., et al., *Coffee consumption and risk of fractures: A systematic review and dose–response meta-analysis.* Bone, 2014. **63**: p. 20-28.

142.   Botelho, F., N. Lunet, and H. Barros, *Coffee and gastric cancer: systematic review and meta-analysis.* Cadernos de Saúde Pública, 2006. **22**: p. 889-900.

143.   Pillay, L., *A Systematic Review: Examining the Relationship Between Coffee Consumption and Breast Cancer.* 2013, Georgia State.

144.   Je, Y., W. Liu, and E. Giovannucci, *Coffee consumption and risk of colorectal cancer: A systematic review and meta-analysis of prospective cohort studies.* International Journal of Cancer, 2009. **124**(7): p. 1662-1668.

145.   Zeegers, M.P., et al., *Are coffee and tea consumption associated with urinary tract cancer risk? A systematic review and meta-analysis.* International Journal of Epidemiology, 2001. **30**(2): p. 353-362.

[212]

146.   Chen, J. and S. Long, *Tea and Coffee Consumption and Risk of Laryngeal Cancer: A Systematic Review Meta-Analysis.* PLoS ONE, 2014. **9**(12): p. e112006.

147.   Panza, F., et al., *Coffee, tea, and caffeine consumption and prevention of late-life cognitive decline and dementia: A systematic review.* The Journal of Nutrition, Health & Aging, 2015. **19**(3): p. 313-328.

148.   Grosso, G., et al., *Coffee, tea, caffeine and risk of depression: a systematic review and dose-response meta-analysis of observational studies.* Molecular Nutrition & Food Research, 2015: p. n/a-n/a.

149.   Zhao, Y., et al., *Association of coffee drinking with all-cause mortality: a systematic review and meta-analysis.* Public Health Nutrition, 2015. **18**(07): p. 1282-1291.

150.   Lowery, L., *Fat*, in *Essentials of Sports Nutrition and Supplements*. 2008, Springer. p. 267-280.

151.   Rona, R.J., et al., *The prevalence of food allergy: A meta-analysis.* Journal of Allergy and Clinical Immunology, 2007. **120**(3): p. 638-646.

152.   Holt, S., J. Miller, and P. Petocz, *An insulin index of foods: the insulin demand generated by 1000-kJ portions of common foods.* The American Journal of Clinical Nutrition, 1997. **66**(5): p. 1264-1276.

153.   Josse, A.R., et al., *Increased consumption of dairy foods and protein during diet- and exercise-induced weight loss promotes fat mass loss and lean mass gain in overweight and obese premenopausal women.* J Nutr, 2011. **141**(9): p. 1626-34.

154.   Zemel, M.B., et al., *Calcium and dairy acceleration of weight and fat loss during energy restriction in obese adults.* Obes Res, 2004. **12**(4): p. 582-90.

155.   Zemel, M.B., et al., *Effects of calcium and dairy on body composition and weight loss in African-American adults.* Obes Res, 2005. **13**(7): p. 1218-25.

156.   Zemel, M.B., *Role of calcium and dairy products in energy partitioning and weight management.* Am J Clin Nutr, 2004. **79**(5): p. 907s-912s.

157.   Abargouei, A.S., et al., *Effect of dairy consumption on weight and body composition in adults: a systematic review and*

meta-analysis of randomized controlled clinical trials. Int J Obes (Lond), 2012. **36**(12): p. 1485-93.

158. Chen, M., et al., *Effects of dairy intake on body weight and fat: a meta-analysis of randomized controlled trials.* Am J Clin Nutr, 2012. **96**(4): p. 735-47.

159. Tong, X., et al., *Dairy consumption and risk of type 2 diabetes mellitus: a meta-analysis of cohort studies.* Eur J Clin Nutr, 2011. **65**(9): p. 1027-31.

160. Gao, D., et al., *Dairy products consumption and risk of type 2 diabetes: systematic review and dose-response meta-analysis.* PLoS One, 2013. **8**(9): p. e73965.

161. Rideout, T.C., et al., *Consumption of low-fat dairy foods for 6 months improves insulin resistance without adversely affecting lipids or bodyweight in healthy adults: a randomized free-living cross-over study.* Nutr J, 2013. **12**: p. 56.

162. Watanabe, F., *Vitamin B12 sources and bioavailability.* Exp Biol Med (Maywood), 2007. **232**(10): p. 1266-74.

163. Watanabe, F., et al., *Vitamin B(12)-Containing Plant Food Sources for Vegetarians.* Nutrients, 2014. **6**(5): p. 1861-1873.

164. National Institutes of Health. *NIH Human Microbiome Project defines normal bacterial makeup of the body.* 2015; Available from: http://www.ncbi.nlm.nih.gov/pubmed/.

165. Biasucci, G., et al., *Cesarean delivery may affect the early biodiversity of intestinal bacteria.* J Nutr, 2008. **138**(9): p. 1796s-1800s.

166. Dominguez-Bello, M.G., et al., *Delivery mode shapes the acquisition and structure of the initial microbiota across multiple body habitats in newborns.* Proc Natl Acad Sci U S A, 2010. **107**(26): p. 11971-5.

167. Gronlund, M.M., et al., *Fecal microflora in healthy infants born by different methods of delivery: permanent changes in intestinal flora after cesarean delivery.* J Pediatr Gastroenterol Nutr, 1999. **28**(1): p. 19-25.

168. Palmer, C., et al., *Development of the human infant intestinal microbiota.* PLoS Biol, 2007. **5**(7): p. e177.

169. Decker, E., et al., *Cesarean delivery is associated with celiac disease but not inflammatory bowel disease in children.* Pediatrics, 2010. **125**(6): p. e1433-40.

[214]

170. Renz-Polster, H., et al., *Caesarean section delivery and the risk of allergic disorders in childhood.* Clin Exp Allergy, 2005. **35**(11): p. 1466-72.

171. Negele, K., et al., *Mode of delivery and development of atopic disease during the first 2 years of life.* Pediatr Allergy Immunol, 2004. **15**(1): p. 48-54.

172. Eggesbo, M., et al., *Is delivery by cesarean section a risk factor for food allergy?* J Allergy Clin Immunol, 2003. **112**(2): p. 420-6.

173. Jost, T., et al., *Impact of human milk bacteria and oligosaccharides on neonatal gut microbiota establishment and gut health.* Nutrition Reviews, 2015. **73**(7): p. 426-437.

174. Jost, T., et al., *Vertical mother-neonate transfer of maternal gut bacteria via breastfeeding.* Environ Microbiol, 2014. **16**(9): p. 2891-904.

175. Holscher, H.D., et al., *Effects of prebiotic-containing infant formula on gastrointestinal tolerance and fecal microbiota in a randomized controlled trial.* JPEN Journal of Parenteral & Enteral Nutrition, 2012. **36**(1 Suppl): p. 95S-105s.

176. Holscher, H.D., et al., *Agave Inulin Supplementation Affects the Fecal Microbiota of Healthy Adults Participating in a Randomized, Double-Blind, Placebo-Controlled, Crossover Trial.* Journal of Nutrition, 2015. **145**(9): p. 2025-2032.

177. Molin, G., *Probiotics in foods not containing milk or milk constituents, with special reference to Lactobacillus plantarum 299v.* Am J Clin Nutr, 2001. **73**(2 Suppl): p. 380S-385S.

178. Fasano, A., *Leaky Gut and Autoimmune Diseases.* Clinical Reviews in Allergy & Immunology, 2012. **42**(1): p. 71-78.

179. Saggioro, A., *Leaky Gut, Microbiota, and Cancer: An Incoming Hypothesis.* Journal of Clinical Gastroenterology, 2014. **48**: p. S62-S66.

180. Luettig, J., et al., *Claudin-2 as a mediator of leaky gut barrier during intestinal inflammation.* Tissue Barriers, 2015. **3**(1-2): p. e977176.

181. Leblhuber, F., et al., *Elevated fecal calprotectin in patients with Alzheimer's dementia indicates leaky gut.* Journal of Neural Transmission, 2015: p. 1-4.

182.   de Kort, S., D. Keszthelyi, and A.A.M. Masclee, *Leaky gut and diabetes mellitus: what is the link?* Obesity Reviews, 2011. **12**(6): p. 449-458.

183.   Reyes, H., et al., *Is a leaky gut involved in the pathogenesis of intrahepatic cholestasis of pregnancy?* Hepatology, 2006. **43**(4): p. 715-722.

184.   Ilan, Y., *Leaky gut and the liver: A role for bacterial translocation in nonalcoholic steatohepatitis.* World Journal of Gastroenterology : WJG, 2012. **18**(21): p. 2609-2618.

185.   Terjung, B. and U. Spengler, *Atypical p-ANCA in PSC and AIH: A Hint Toward a "leaky gut"?* Clinical Reviews in Allergy & Immunology, 2009. **36**(1): p. 40-51.

186.   Hartmann, P., W.-C. Chen, and B. Schnabl, *The intestinal microbiome and the leaky gut as therapeutic targets in alcoholic liver disease.* Frontiers in Physiology, 2012. **3**: p. 402.

187.   Lepper, P.M., et al. *Association of lipopolysaccharide-binding protein and coronary artery disease in men.* J Am Coll Cardiol, 2007. **50**(1): p. 25-31.

188.   Moran, A.P., M.M. Prendergast, and B.J. Appelmelk, *Molecular mimicry of host structures by bacterial lipopolysaccharides and its contribution to disease.* FEMS Immunol Med Microbiol, 1996. **16**(2): p. 105-15.

189.   Chastain, E.M. and S.D. Miller, *Molecular mimicry as an inducing trigger for CNS autoimmune demyelinating disease.* Immunol Rev, 2012. **245**(1): p. 227-38.

190.   Maes, M., M. Kubera, and J.C. Leunis, *The gut-brain barrier in major depression: intestinal mucosal dysfunction with an increased translocation of LPS from gram negative enterobacteria (leaky gut) plays a role in the inflammatory pathophysiology of depression.* Neuro Endocrinol Lett, 2008. **29**(1): p. 117-24.

191.   Cani, P.D., et al., *Metabolic endotoxemia initiates obesity and insulin resistance.* Diabetes, 2007. **56**(7): p. 1761-72.

192.   Fei, N. and L. Zhao, *An opportunistic pathogen isolated from the gut of an obese human causes obesity in germfree mice.* Isme j, 2013. **7**(4): p. 880-4.

193.   Moreno-Navarrete, J.M., et al., *Circulating lipopolysaccharide-binding protein (LBP) as a marker of obesity-related insulin resistance.* Int J Obes (Lond), 2012. **36**(11): p. 1442-9.

194. Ruiz, A.G., et al., *Lipopolysaccharide-binding protein plasma levels and liver TNF-alpha gene expression in obese patients: evidence for the potential role of endotoxin in the pathogenesis of non-alcoholic steatohepatitis.* Obes Surg, 2007. **17**(10): p. 1374-80.

195. Plaza-Díaz, J., et al., *Pyrosequencing Analysis Reveals Changes in Intestinal Microbiota of Healthy Adults Who Received a Daily Dose of Immunomodulatory Probiotic Strains.* Nutrients, 2015. **7**(6): p. 3999-4015.

196. Nylund, L., et al., *Microarray analysis reveals marked intestinal microbiota aberrancy in infants having eczema compared to healthy children in at-risk for atopic disease.* BMC Microbiology, 2013. **13**(1): p. 1-11.

197. Valentini, L., et al., *Impact of personalized diet and probiotic supplementation on inflammation, nutritional parameters and intestinal microbiota – The "RISTOMED project": Randomized controlled trial in healthy older people.* Clinical Nutrition, 2015. **34**(4): p. 593-602.

198. Rampelli, S., et al., *A probiotics-containing biscuit modulates the intestinal microbiota in the elderly.* Journal of Nutrition, Health & Aging, 2013. **17**(2): p. 166-172.

199. Ukena, S.N., et al., *Probiotic <italic>Escherichia coli</italic> Nissle 1917 Inhibits Leaky Gut by Enhancing Mucosal Integrity.* PLoS ONE, 2007. **2**(12): p. e1308.

200. Zhong, W., et al., *Dietary niacin supplementation ameliorates ethanol-induced liver injury in rats through sealing the leaky gut.* The FASEB Journal, 2012. **26**(1_MeetingAbstracts): p. lb765.

201. Maes, M. and J.-C. Leunis, *Normalization of leaky gut in chronic fatigue syndrome (CFS) is accompanied by a clinical improvement: effects of age, duration of illness and the translocation of LPS from gram-negative bacteria.* Neuro Endocrinology Lett, 2008. **29**(6): p. 902-910.

202. Sturniolo, G.C., et al., *Zinc supplementation tightens "Leaky Gut" in Crohn's disease.* Inflammatory Bowel Diseases, 2001. **7**(2): p. 94-98.

203. Kassam, Z., et al., *Fecal microbiota transplantation for Clostridium difficile infection: systematic review and meta-*

analysis. The American Journal Of Gastroenterology, 2013. **108**(4): p. 500-508.

204.   Rossen, N.G., et al., *Fecal microbiota transplantation as novel therapy in gastroenterology: A systematic review.* World Journal Of Gastroenterology: WJG, 2015. **21**(17): p. 5359-5371.

205.   Colman, R.J. and D.T. Rubin, *Fecal microbiota transplantation as therapy for inflammatory bowel disease: a systematic review and meta-analysis.* Journal Of Crohn's & Colitis, 2014. **8**(12): p. 1569-1581.

206.   Benton, D., R. Griffiths, and J. Haller, *Thiamine supplementation mood and cognitive functioning.* Psychopharmacology (Berl), 1997. **129**: p. 66-71.

207.   Schoenen, J., J. Jacquy, and M. Lenaerts, *Effectiveness of high-dose riboflavin in migraine prophylaxis A randomized controlled trial.* Neurology, 1998. **50**(2): p. 466-470.

208.   Albertson, A., et al., *Nutrient intakes of 2-to 10-year-old American children: 10-year trends.* Journal of the American Dietetic Association, 1992. **92**(12): p. 1492-1496.

209.   Ashokkumar, B., et al., *Effect of folate oversupplementation on folate uptake by human intestinal and renal epithelial cells.* The American Journal of Clinical Nutrition, 2007. **86**(1): p. 159-166.

210.   Kelly, P., et al., *Unmetabolized folic acid in serum: acute studies in subjects consuming fortified food and supplements.* The American Journal of Clinical Nutrition, 1997. **65**(6): p. 1790-1795.

211.   Smith, A.D., Y.-I. Kim, and H. Refsum, *Is folic acid good for everyone?* The American Journal of Clinical Nutrition, 2008. **87**(3): p. 517-533.

212.   Wright, A.J., J.R. Dainty, and P.M. Finglas, *Folic acid metabolism in human subjects revisited: potential implications for proposed mandatory folic acid fortification in the UK.* British Journal of Nutrition, 2007. **98**(04): p. 667-675.

213.   Troen, A.M., et al., *Unmetabolized folic acid in plasma is associated with reduced natural killer cell cytotoxicity among postmenopausal women.* The Journal of Nutrition, 2006. **136**(1): p. 189-194.

214. Hemila, H. and E. Chalker, *Vitamin C for preventing and treating the common cold.* Cochrane Database Syst Rev, 2013. **1**: p. CD000980.

215. Huang, H.-Y. and L.J. Appel, *Supplementation of Diets with α-Tocopherol Reduces Serum Concentrations of γ- and δ-Tocopherol in Humans.* The Journal of Nutrition, 2003. **133**(10): p. 3137-3140.

216. Taubert, K., *[Magnesium in migraine. Results of a multicenter pilot study].* Fortschr Med, 1994. **112**: p. 328-30.

217. Peikert, A., C. Wilimzig, and R. Kohne-Volland, *Prophylaxis of migraine with oral magnesium: results from a prospective, multi-center, placebo-controlled and double-blind randomized study.* Cephalalgia, 1996. **16**: p. 257-63.

218. Facchinetti, F., et al., *Magnesium prophylaxis of menstrual migraine: effects on intracellular magnesium.* Headache, 1991. **31**: p. 298-301.

219. Wang, F., et al., *Oral magnesium oxide prophylaxis of frequent migrainous headache in children: a randomized, double-blind, placebo-controlled trial.* Headache, 2003. **43**: p. 601-10.

220. Attias, J., et al., *Oral magnesium intake reduces permanent hearing loss induced by noise exposure.* Am J Otolaryngol, 1994. **15**: p. 26-32.

221. Sanjuliani, A.F., V.G. de Abreu Fagundes, and E.A. Francischetti, *Effects of magnesium on blood pressure and intracellular ion levels of Brazilian hypertensive patients*, in *Int J Cardiol*. 1996: Ireland. p. 177-83.

222. Guerrero-Romero, F. and M. Rodriguez-Moran, *The effect of lowering blood pressure by magnesium supplementation in diabetic hypertensive adults with low serum magnesium levels: a randomized, double-blind, placebo-controlled clinical trial.* J Hum Hypertens, 2009. **23**: p. 245-51.

223. Witteman, J.C., et al., *Reduction of blood pressure with oral magnesium supplementation in women with mild to moderate hypertension.* Am J Clin Nutr, 1994. **60**: p. 129-35.

224. Fontana-Klaiber, H. and B. Hogg, *[Therapeutic effects of magnesium in dysmenorrhea].* Schweiz Rundsch Med Prax, 1990. **79**: p. 491-4.

225.   Seifert, B., et al., *[Magnesium--a new therapeutic alternative in primary dysmenorrhea].* Zentralbl Gynakol, 1989. **111**: p. 755-60.

226.   De Souza, M.C., et al., *A synergistic effect of a daily supplement for 1 month of 200 mg magnesium plus 50 mg vitamin B6 for the relief of anxiety-related premenstrual symptoms: a randomized, double-blind, crossover study.* J Womens Health Gend Based Med, 2000. **9**: p. 131-9.

227.   Facchinetti, F., et al., *Oral magnesium successfully relieves premenstrual mood changes.* Obstet Gynecol, 1991. **78**: p. 177-81.

228.   Barel, A., et al., *Effect of oral intake of choline-stabilized orthosilicic acid on skin, nails and hair in women with photodamaged skin.* Arch Dermatol Res, 2005. **297**: p. 147-53.

229.   Whelton, P.K., et al., *Effects of oral potassium on blood pressure: Meta-analysis of randomized controlled clinical trials.* JAMA, 1997. **277**(20): p. 1624-1632.

230.   Singh, M. and R.R. Das, *Zinc for the common cold.* Cochrane Database Syst Rev, 2015.

231.   Lazzerini, M. and L. Ronfani, *Oral zinc for treating diarrhoea in children.* Cochrane Database Syst Rev, 2013.

232.   Bilici, M., et al., *Double-blind, placebo-controlled study of zinc sulfate in the treatment of attention deficit hyperactivity disorder.* Prog Neuropsychopharmacol Biol Psychiatry, 2004. **28**: p. 181-90.

233.   Delgado-Lista, J., et al., *Long chain omega-3 fatty acids and cardiovascular disease: a systematic review.* British Journal of Nutrition, 2012. **107**(SupplementS2): p. S201-S213.

234.   Montori, V.M., et al., *Fish oil supplementation in type 2 diabetes: a quantitative systematic review.* Diabetes Care, 2000. **23**(9): p. 1407-1415.

235.   Eslick, G.D., et al., *Benefits of fish oil supplementation in hyperlipidemia: a systematic review and meta-analysis.* International Journal of Cardiology, 2009. **136**(1): p. 4-16.

236.   Balk, E.M., et al., *Effects of omega-3 fatty acids on serum markers of cardiovascular disease risk: A systematic review.* Atherosclerosis, 2006. **189**(1): p. 19-30.

237. Campbell, F., et al., *A systematic review of fish-oil supplements for the prevention and treatment of hypertension.* European Journal of Preventive Cardiology, 2013. **20**(1): p. 107-120.

238. Wang, C., et al., *n−3 Fatty acids from fish or fish-oil supplements, but not α-linolenic acid, benefit cardiovascular disease outcomes in primary- and secondary-prevention studies: a systematic review.* The American Journal of Clinical Nutrition, 2006. **84**(1): p. 5-17.

239. León, H., et al., *Effect of fish oil on arrhythmias and mortality: systematic review.* BMJ, 2008. **337**.

240. Rizos, E.C., et al., *Association between omega-3 fatty acid supplementation and risk of major cardiovascular disease events: A systematic review and meta-analysis.* JAMA, 2012. **308**(10): p. 1024-1033.

241. Wendland, E., et al., *Effect of α linolenic acid on cardiovascular risk markers: a systematic review.* Heart, 2006. **92**(2): p. 166-169.

242. Appleton, K.M., P.J. Rogers, and A.R. Ness, *Updated systematic review and meta-analysis of the effects of n−3 long-chain polyunsaturated fatty acids on depressed mood.* The American Journal of Clinical Nutrition, 2010.

243. Appleton, K.M., et al., *Effects of n−3 long-chain polyunsaturated fatty acids on depressed mood: systematic review of published trials.* The American Journal of Clinical Nutrition, 2006. **84**(6): p. 1308-1316.

244. Miles, E.A. and P.C. Calder, *Influence of marine n-3 polyunsaturated fatty acids on immune function and a systematic review of their effects on clinical outcomes in rheumatoid arthritis.* British Journal of Nutrition, 2012. **107**(SupplementS2): p. S171-S184.

245. Schuchardt, J.P., et al., *Incorporation of EPA and DHA into plasma phospholipids in response to different omega-3 fatty acid formulations--a comparative bioavailability study of fish oil vs. krill oil.* Lipids Health Dis, 2011. **10**: p. 145.

246. Ulven, S., et al., *Metabolic Effects of Krill Oil are Essentially Similar to Those of Fish Oil but at Lower Dose of EPA and DHA, in Healthy Volunteers.* Lipids, 2011. **46**(1): p. 37-46.

247. Tang, G., et al., *Short-term (intestinal) and long-term (postintestinal) conversion of β-carotene to retinol in adults as*

assessed by a stable-isotope reference method. The American Journal of Clinical Nutrition, 2003. **78**(2): p. 259-266.

248.   Wang, J., et al., *Vitamin A equivalence of spirulina ß-carotene in Chinese adults as assessed by using a stable-isotope reference method.* The American Journal of Clinical Nutrition, 2008. **87**(6): p. 1730-1737.

249.   Tang, G., et al., *Golden Rice is an effective source of vitamin A.* The American Journal of Clinical Nutrition, 2009. **89**(6): p. 1776-1783.

250.   *Vitamin B12 Deficiency.* New England Journal of Medicine, 2013. **368**(21): p. 2040-2042.

251.   Freeman, A.G., *Cyanocobalamin--a case for withdrawal: discussion paper.* Journal of the Royal Society of Medicine, 1992. **85**(11): p. 686-687.

252.   Matte, J.J., F. Guay, and C.L. Girard, *Bioavailability of vitamin B12 in cows' milk.* British Journal of Nutrition, 2012. **107**(01): p. 61-66.

253.   Koyama, K., et al., *Efficacy of methylcobalamin on lowering total homocysteine plasma concentrations in haemodialysis patients receiving high-dose folic acid supplementation.* Nephrology Dialysis Transplantation, 2002. **17**(5): p. 916-922.

254.   Pfohl-Leszkowicz, A., G. Keith, and G. Dirheimer, *Effect of cobalamin derivatives on in vitro enzymic DNA methylation: methylcobalamin can act as a methyl donor.* Biochemistry, 1991. **30**(32): p. 8045-8051.

255.   Campbell, B., et al., *International Society of Sports Nutrition position stand: protein and exercise.* Journal of the International Society of Sports Nutrition, 2007. **4**: p. 8-8.

256.   Helms, E.R., A.A. Aragon, and P.J. Fitschen, *Evidence-based recommendations for natural bodybuilding contest preparation: nutrition and supplementation.* Journal of the International Society of Sports Nutrition, 2014. **11**: p. 20-20.

257.   Antonio, J., et al., *A high protein diet (3.4 g/kg/d) combined with a heavy resistance training program improves body composition in healthy trained men and women – a follow-up investigation.* Journal of the International Society of Sports Nutrition, 2015. **12**: p. 39.

258. Antonio, J., et al., *Essentials of Sports Nutrition and Supplements.* 2009, New York, USA: Springer Science & Business Media.

259. Last, A.R. and S.A. Wilson, *Low-carbohydrate diets.* Am Fam Physician, 2006. **73**(11): p. 1951-1958.

260. Westman, E.C., et al., *Low-carbohydrate nutrition and metabolism.* The American Journal of Clinical Nutrition, 2007. **86**(2): p. 276-284.

261. Hu, T., et al., *Effects of Low-Carbohydrate Diets Versus Low-Fat Diets on Metabolic Risk Factors: A Meta-Analysis of Randomized Controlled Clinical Trials.* American Journal of Epidemiology, 2012. **176**(suppl 7): p. S44-S54.

262. Wood, R.J. and M.L. Fernandez, *Carbohydrate-restricted versus low-glycemic-index diets for the treatment of insulin resistance and metabolic syndrome.* Nutr Rev, 2009. **67**(3): p. 179-183.

263. Hamilton, J.A., *Fatty acid transport: difficult or easy?* Journal of Lipid Research, 1998. **39**(3): p. 467-481.

264. Schonfeld, P. and G. Reiser, *Why does brain metabolism not favor burning of fatty acids to provide energy[quest] - Reflections on disadvantages of the use of free fatty acids as fuel for brain.* J Cereb Blood Flow Metab, 2013. **33**(10): p. 1493-1499.

265. Kaleta, C., et al., *In Silico Evidence for Gluconeogenesis from Fatty Acids in Humans.* PLoS Computational Biology, 2011. **7**(7): p. e1002116.

266. Lefevre, F. and N. Aronson, *Ketogenic Diet for the Treatment of Refractory Epilepsy in Children: A Systematic Review of Efficacy.* Pediatrics, 2000. **105**(4): p. e46.

267. Keene, D.L., *A Systematic Review of the Use of the Ketogenic Diet in Childhood Epilepsy.* Pediatric Neurology, 2006. **35**(1): p. 1-5.

268. Levy, R.G., et al., *Ketogenic diet and other dietary treatments for epilepsy.* The Cochrane Library, 2012.

269. Henderson, C.B., et al., *Efficacy of the Ketogenic Diet as a Treatment Option for Epilepsy: Meta-analysis.* Journal of Child Neurology, 2006. **21**(3): p. 193-198.

270.   Neal, E.G., et al., *The ketogenic diet for the treatment of childhood epilepsy: a randomised controlled trial.* The Lancet Neurology, 2008. **7**(6): p. 500-506.

271.   Kossoff, E.H., et al., *A randomized, crossover comparison of daily carbohydrate limits using the modified Atkins diet.* Epilepsy & Behavior, 2007. **10**(3): p. 432-436.

272.   Kossoff, E.H., et al., *A prospective study of the modified Atkins diet for intractable epilepsy in adults.* Epilepsia, 2008. **49**(2): p. 316-319.

273.   Freeman, J.M., *The ketogenic diet: a treatment for children and others with epilepsy.* 2007: Demos medical publishing.

274.   Huttenlocher, P., A. Wilbourn, and J. Signore, *Medium-chain triglycerides as a therapy for intractable childhood epilepsy.* Neurology, 1971. **21**(11): p. 1097-1097.

275.   Trauner, D.A., *Medium-chain triglyceride (MCT) diet in intractable seizure disorders.* Neurology, 1985. **35**(2): p. 237.

276.   Huttenlocher, P.R., *Ketonemia and Seizures: Metabolic and Anticonvulsant Effects of Two Ketogenic Diets in Childhood Epilepsy.* Pediatr Res, 1976. **10**(5): p. 536-540.

277.   Royer, P., *Periodic functional ketosis in children.* Vie médicale (Paris, France: 1920), 1954. **35**(1): p. 9.

278.   Sargent, F., et al., *THE EFFECTS OF ENVIRONMENT AND OTHER FACTORS ON NUTRITIONAL KETOSIS.* Quarterly Journal of Experimental Physiology and Cognate Medical Sciences, 1958. **43**(4): p. 345-351.

279.   Krebs, H., *Biochemical aspects of ketosis.* Proceedings of the Royal Society of Medicine, 1960. **53**(2): p. 71.

280.   Krebs, H.A., *The regulation of the release of ketone bodies by the liver.* Advances in Enzyme Regulation, 1966. **4**(0): p. 339-353.

281.   Volek, J.S. and S.D. Phinney, *The Art and Science of Low Carbohydrate Living: Beyond Obesity.* 2013, New York, USA: Beyond Obesity.

282.   Volek, J.S. and S.D. Phinney, *LOW CARBOHYDRATE LIVING.* 2011, New York, USA: Beyond Obesity.

283.   Chul Kang, H., et al., *Efficacy and Safety of the Ketogenic Diet for Intractable Childhood Epilepsy: Korean Multicentric Experience.* Epilepsia, 2005. **46**(2): p. 272-279.

284. Kang, H.-C., et al., *Safe and Effective Use of the Ketogenic Diet in Children with Epilepsy and Mitochondrial Respiratory Chain Complex Defects.* Epilepsia, 2007. **48**(1): p. 82-88.

285. Suo, C., et al., *Efficacy and safety of the ketogenic diet in Chinese children.* Seizure - European Journal of Epilepsy. **22**(3): p. 174-178.

286. Lyczkowski, D.A., et al., *Safety and Tolerability of the Ketogenic Diet in Pediatric Epilepsy: Effects of Valproate Combination Therapy.* Epilepsia, 2005. **46**(9): p. 1533-1538.

287. Dressler, A., et al., *Type 1 diabetes and epilepsy: Efficacy and safety of the ketogenic diet.* Epilepsia, 2010. **51**(6): p. 1086-1089.

288. Kossoff, E.H., et al., *Efficacy of the Ketogenic Diet for Infantile Spasms.* Pediatrics, 2002. **109**(5): p. 780-783.

289. Guo, C., et al., *[A clinical trial of ketogenic diet in patients with acute spinal cord injury: safety and feasibility].* Nan fang yi ke da xue xue bao = Journal of Southern Medical University, 2014. **34**(4): p. 571-575.

290. Fine, E.J., et al., *Targeting insulin inhibition as a metabolic therapy in advanced cancer: A pilot safety and feasibility dietary trial in 10 patients.* Nutrition, 2012. **28**(10): p. 1028-1035.

291. Rieger, J., et al., *The ERGO trial: A pilot study of a ketogenic diet in patients with recurrent glioblastoma.* J Clin Oncol (Meeting Abstracts), 2010. **28**(15_suppl): p. e12532-.

292. Schmidt, M., et al., *Effects of a ketogenic diet on the quality of life in 16 patients with advanced cancer: A pilot trial.* Nutr Metab (Lond), 2011. **8**(1): p. 54.

293. Yancy, J.W.S., et al., *A Low-Carbohydrate, Ketogenic Diet versus a Low-Fat Diet To Treat Obesity and HyperlipidemiaA Randomized, Controlled Trial.* Annals of Internal Medicine, 2004. **140**(10): p. 769-777.

294. Yancy Jr, W.S., et al., *A low-carbohydrate, ketogenic diet to treat type 2 diabetes.* Nutr Metab (Lond), 2005. **2**: p. 34.

295. Sharman, M.J., et al., *A Ketogenic Diet Favorably Affects Serum Biomarkers for Cardiovascular Disease in Normal-Weight Men.* The Journal of Nutrition, 2002. **132**(7): p. 1879-1885.

296.   Kitabchi, A.E., et al., *Hyperglycemic Crises in Adult Patients With Diabetes.* Diabetes Care, 2009. **32**(7): p. 1335-1343.

297.   Thurston, J.H., R.E. Hauhart, and J.A. Schiro, *Beta-hydroxybutyrate reverses insulin-induced hypoglycemic coma in suckling-weanling mice despite low blood and brain glucose levels.* Metab Brain Dis, 1986. **1**(1): p. 63-82.

298.   Owen, O.E., et al., *Brain Metabolism during Fasting*.* The Journal of Clinical Investigation, 1967. **46**(10): p. 1589-1595.

299.   Izumi, Y., et al., *beta-Hydroxybutyrate fuels synaptic function during development. Histological and physiological evidence in rat hippocampal slices.* J Clin Invest, 1998. **101**(5): p. 1121-32.

300.   Henderson, S.T., *High carbohydrate diets and Alzheimer's disease.* Med Hypotheses, 2004. **62**: p. 689-700.

301.   Vanitallie, T.B., et al., *Treatment of Parkinson disease with diet-induced hyperketonemia: a feasibility study.* Neurology, 2005. **64**: p. 728-30.

302.   de Lau, L.M., et al., *Dietary fatty acids and the risk of Parkinson disease: the Rotterdam study.* Neurology, 2005. **64**: p. 2040-5.

303.   Dietitians New Zealand, *Low Carbohydrate High Fat Diet Position Statement.* Dietitians New Zealand, 2014.

304.   Yancy, W.S., Jr., et al., *A Low-Carbohydrate, Ketogenic Diet versus a Low-Fat Diet To Treat Obesity and Hyperlipidemia: A Randomized, Controlled Trial.* Annals of Internal Medicine, 2004. **140**(10): p. 769-77.

305.   Bueno, N.B., et al., *Very-low-carbohydrate ketogenic diet v. low-fat diet for long-term weight loss: a meta-analysis of randomised controlled trials.* British Journal of Nutrition, 2013. **110**(07): p. 1178-1187.

306.   Volek, J.S., E.E. Quann, and C.E. Forsythe, *Low-Carbohydrate Diets Promote a More Favorable Body Composition Than Low-Fat Diets.* Strength and Conditioning Journal, 2010. **32**(1): p. 42-47.

307.   Sondike, S.B., N. Copperman, and M.S. Jacobson, *Effects of a low-carbohydrate diet on weight loss and cardiovascular risk factor in overweight adolescents.* The Journal of Pediatrics, 2003. **142**(3): p. 253-258.

308.   Nordmann, A.J., et al., *Effects of low-carbohydrate vs low-fat diets on weight loss and cardiovascular risk factors: a meta-*

analysis of randomized controlled trials. Arch Intern Med, 2006. **166**(3): p. 285-93.

309.   Dashti, H., et al., *Beneficial effects of ketogenic diet in obese diabetic subjects.* Molecular and Cellular Biochemistry, 2007. **302**(1-2): p. 249-256.

310.   Hussain, T.A., et al., *Effect of low-calorie versus low-carbohydrate ketogenic diet in type 2 diabetes.* Nutrition, 2012. **28**(10): p. 1016-1021.

311.   Nielsen, J.V. and E.A. Joensson, *Low-carbohydrate diet in type 2 diabetes: stable improvement of bodyweight and glycemic control during 44 months follow-up.* Nutr Metab (Lond), 2008. **5**: p. 14.

312.   Warburg, O., *On the origin of cancer cells.* Science, 1956. **123**(3191): p. 309-314.

313.   Seyfried, T.N., et al., *Metabolic therapy: A new paradigm for managing malignant brain cancer.* Cancer Letters, 2015. **356**(2, Part A): p. 289-300.

314.   Bozzetti, F. and B. Zupec-Kania, *Toward a cancer-specific diet.* Clinical Nutrition, 2015 (0).

315.   Vidali, S., et al., *Mitochondria: The ketogenic diet—A metabolism-based therapy.* The International Journal of Biochemistry & Cell Biology, 2015(0).

316.   Napoli, E., N. Dueñas, and C. Giulivi, *Potential therapeutic use of the ketogenic diet in autism spectrum disorders.* Frontiers in Pediatrics, 2014. **2**.

317.   Evangeliou, A., et al., *Application of a ketogenic diet in children with autistic behavior: pilot study.* Journal of Child Neurology, 2003. **18**(2): p. 113-118.

318.   He, Y., et al., *The Transcriptional Repressor DEC2 Regulates Sleep Length in Mammals.* Science (New York, N.Y.), 2009. **325**(5942): p. 866-870.

319.   Hirshkowitz, M., et al., *National Sleep Foundation's sleep time duration recommendations: methodology and results summary.* Sleep Health: Journal of the National Sleep Foundation. **1**(1): p. 40-43.

320.   Ulrich, C.M. and J.D. Potter, *Folate supplementation: too much of a good thing?* Cancer Epidemiology Biomarkers & Prevention, 2006. **15**(2): p. 189-193.

321. Pietrzik, K., L. Bailey, and B. Shane, *Folic acid and L-5-methyltetrahydrofolate.* Clinical Pharmacokinetics, 2010. **49**(8): p. 535-548.

322. Konings, E.J., et al., *Folate intake of the Dutch population according to newly established liquid chromatography data for foods.* The American Journal of Clinical Nutrition, 2001. **73**(4): p. 765-776.

323. Galley, P. and M. Thiollet, *A double-blind, placebo-controlled trial of a new veno-active flavonoid fraction (S 5682) in the treatment of symptomatic capillary fragility.* International Angiology: a journal of the International Union of Angiology, 1993. **12**(1): p. 69-72.

324. Heinrich, U., et al., *Long-term ingestion of high flavanol cocoa provides photoprotection against UV-induced erythema and improves skin condition in women.* J Nutr, 2006. **136**: p. 1565-9.

325. Christie, S., et al., *Flavonoid supplement improves leg health and reduces fluid retention in pre-menopausal women in a double-blind, placebo-controlled study.* Phytomedicine, 2004. **11**: p. 11-7.

326. Board, E.C.R., *Oligomeric Proanthocyanidins.* Natural Therapies Database, 2015.

327. Castell, J.V., et al., *Intestinal absorption of undegraded proteins in men: presence of bromelain in plasma after oral intake.* Am J Physiol, 1997. **273**: p. G139-46.

328. Taussig, S.J. and S. Batkin, *Bromelain, the enzyme complex of pineapple (Ananas comosus) and its clinical application. An update.* Journal of Ethnopharmacology, 1988. **22**(2): p. 191-203.

329. Bernaola Aponte, G., et al., *Probiotics for treating persistent diarrhoea in children.* Cochrane Database Syst Rev, 2015.

330. Allen, S.J., et al., *Probiotics for treating acute infectious diarrhoea.* Cochrane Database Syst Rev, 2010.

331. Johnston, B.C., et al., *Probiotics for the prevention of pediatric antibiotic-associated diarrhea.* Cochrane Database Syst Rev, 2011.

332. Goldenberg, J.Z., et al., *Probiotics for the prevention of Clostridium difficile-associated diarrhea in adults and children.* Cochrane Database Syst Rev. , 2013.

333. Hao, Q., B.R. Dong, and T. Wu, *Probiotics for preventing acute upper respiratory tract infections.* Cochrane Database Syst Rev., 2015.

334. Ramkumar, D. and S.S.C. Rao, *Efficacy and Safety of Traditional Medical Therapies for Chronic Constipation: Systematic Review.* Am J Gastroenterol, 2005. **100**(4): p. 936-971.

335. Bijkerk, C.J., et al., *Systematic review: the role of different types of fibre in the treatment of irritable bowel syndrome.* Alimentary Pharmacology & Therapeutics, 2004. **19**(3): p. 245-251.

336. Suares, N.C. and A.C. Ford, *Systematic review: the effects of fibre in the management of chronic idiopathic constipation.* Alimentary Pharmacology & Therapeutics, 2011. **33**(8): p. 895-901.

337. Merchant, R.E. and C.A. Andre, *A review of recent clinical trials of the nutritional supplement Chlorella pyrenoidosa in the treatment of fibromyalgia, hypertension, and ulcerative colitis.* Altern Ther Health Med, 2001. **7**: p. 79-91.

338. Mathew, B., et al., *Evaluation of chemoprevention of oral cancer with Spirulina fusiformis.* Nutr Cancer, 1995. **24**: p. 197-202.

339. Cingi, C., et al., *The effects of spirulina on allergic rhinitis.* Eur Arch Otorhinolaryngol, 2008. **265**: p. 1219-23.

340. Mao, T.K., J. Van de Water, and M.E. Gershwin, *Effects of a Spirulina-based dietary supplement on cytokine production from allergic rhinitis patients.* J Med Food, 2005. **8**: p. 27-30.

341. Roza, A.M. and H.M. Shizgal, *The Harris Benedict equation reevaluated: resting energy requirements and the body cell mass.* The American Journal of Clinical Nutrition, 1984. **40**(1): p. 168-182.

-